77 Body Weight and Dumbbell Exercises for Seniors

A Guide to Safe and Effective Strength Training and Workouts to Improve Stability, Posture, and Wellbeing Over 60

Andy Taumann

© Copyright 2022 Andy Taumann - All Rights Reserved

Published by Andy Taumann

Th.-Heuss Str. 25, 96215 Lichtenfels, Germany

andreas.taumann@web.de

Legal Notice

This book is copyright protected and for personal use only. You cannot reproduce, duplicate, transmit, amend, distribute, sell, use, quote, or perpetuate any part or the content within this book without the direct consent of the author or publisher.

Disclaimer

By reading this book, you accept this disclaimer in full. The information provided within this book is for general informational purposes only. Even though it has been attempted to present accurate information, there are no representations or warranties, express or implied, about the completeness, accuracy, or reliability of the information, products, services, or related graphics contained in this book for any purpose. The information is provided "as is," to be used at your own risk. The author is not a medical professional and nothing in this publication constitutes medical advice. Any exercise program, including the exercise routines outlined in this publication, may result in injury. The author will not assume any liability for direct or indirect losses or damages that may result from the use of information contained in this book including but not limited to economic loss, injury, illness, or death. To reduce the risk of injury, consult your doctor before beginning any exercise program. The information in this book is meant to supplement, not replace, proper hypertrophy training. Like any sport involving speed, equipment, balance, and environmental factors, weight training poses some inherent risk. The author and publisher advise readers to take full responsibility for their safety and know their limits. Before practicing the skills described in this book, be sure that your equipment is well maintained and do not take risks beyond your level of experience, aptitude, training, and comfort level. All trademarks appearing in this book are the property of their respective owners.

Table of Contents

Introduction 9

Why Seniors Should Work Out 12

Workout Fundamentals for Seniors 14

    General Programming Basics 15

    Senior Specific Training Advice 18

77 Body Weight and Dumbbell Exercises for Seniors 23

    Main Muscles of the Body - Front 25

    Main Muscles of the Body - Back 26

    Shoulders 27

    Back 43

    Chest 50

    Biceps 61

    Triceps 66

    Forearms 74

    Abs 80

    Quads 89

    Glutes and Hamstrings 101

    Calves 110

Example Programs 115

    Template 1 - 2-Day-Program 118

    Template 2 - 3-Day-Program 119

    Template 3 - 4-Day-Program 120

    2-Day Beginner Program (without bench) 121

    2-Day Beginner Program (with bench) 122

    3-Day Beginner Program (without bench) 123

    3-Day Beginner Program (with bench) 124

    3-Day Intermediate Program (without bench) 125

    3-Day Intermediate Program (with bench) 126

    4-Day Intermediate Program (without bench) 127

    4-Day Intermediate Program (with bench) 128

    Adapting and Developing a Program 129

Conclusion 130

References 131

Introduction

Hello and welcome to *"77 Body Weight and Dumbbell Exercises for Seniors - A Guide to Safe and Effective Strength Training and Workouts to Improve Stability, Posture, and Wellbeing Over 60"*! Before we begin, I would like to thank you from the bottom of my heart for your purchase and the trust you have placed in me. It really means a lot, and I hope that I will not disappoint you with the exercises presented in this book. I have tried to tailor this book as closely as possible to the training needs and potential goals of seniors like you to give you the tools to live (or keep living) a strong, healthy, and independent life.

My name is Andy. I am a 33-year-old passionate lifter who has learned a lot about this sport over the years and now wishes to share his knowledge with you. Having injury-prone shoulders and knees (which both needed several surgeries in the past) and a notoriously weak bone and joint structure, weight training is one of the few sports that I can still safely perform. Thankfully, it also allowed me to personally experience the many benefits it brings. It helped me alleviate many of my joint issues by making me stronger and more resistant to injury - and got me in decent shape if I may say so myself. Of course, finding the right exercises to accomplish this was easier said than done. After all, there were dozens and dozens of influencers, physical therapists, and strength coaches out there who all seemed to recommend or condemn something different. However, in the end, I found that the choice of exercise highly depended on the individual. What matters for any person who wants to train, old or young, is finding exercises that work for them and allow them to get stronger without causing pain or discomfort - which leads us neatly to this book.

I firmly believe that strength training is one of the best things anyone can do for their body. I also believe that no one needs strength training more than seniors or the elderly because it might very well change their lives. In fact, this conviction is part of the reason why I wrote this book.

Apart from training for my own longevity, there is also a senior in my life who is very close to me but, sadly, very unhealthy and overweight. They have never cared much about their health, let alone exercising, and no matter how much I encourage and preach, they are just too stubborn and set in their ways to listen. This person has just turned seventy, but already has issues with seemingly mundane tasks like taking the stairs, walking a couple of hundred yards, getting out of an armchair, or picking up something from the floor. Sadly, despite these ever-increasing limitations, they don't want to hear anything about exercising. They would rather stay in their comfort zone, even though just a little weight training - just a little effort - would yield infinite returns on their quality of life.

I accepted that I may not be able to help this person. But I may be able to help you because you still want to listen. You still want to make a change for the better. Let me tell you how much I respect that because I know all too well that not everyone has this kind of will and courage.

That's why this book contains all there is to know about getting and staying strong and fit at home as you get older.

We begin with a short summary of all the benefits that strength training has in store for you and follow up with tried-and-tested training principles for muscle strength and growth. After all, I figured it wouldn't be particularly useful to merely show you a few exercises without telling you how to apply them in a program. However, since many older people need to watch out for different things in their training than younger people, I also adapted these training principles to the needs and goals of seniors.

After we have covered this, we delve into the actual exercises and see how we can apply them in some example programs for both beginners and intermediates. Ability can vary greatly among seniors, from highly robust people, who maybe want to take preventive measures to preserve their strength, to more frail people with possible limitations, who need to approach exercising more carefully and thoughtfully. For that reason, I tried to include exercises and programs for both of these and everyone in between.

Of course, aside from strength training, cardio training and nutrition also play a vital role for seniors to achieve maximum health benefits. These may be outside the scope of this book, but it would be remiss not to at least mention them.

After all, doing some light and joint-friendly cardio activities like walking, swimming, or cycling for maybe 20-30 minutes a day will help further strengthen your arguably most important muscle - your heart. Combining this with a varied, protein-rich diet consisting mostly of whole foods, fruits, vegetables, fish, lean meats, and healthy dairy products will probably be optimal.

Still, even strength training alone might already work wonders for your health. I hope that after reading this book and applying its principles you will see this for yourself. If you do, might I be so bold as to ask a small favor of you? If you could spare just a minute of your time, could you please leave an honest review on Amazon to share your opinion and experience? Your feedback is valuable to me, and I would highly appreciate it.

As a final side note, please know that English is my second language. I therefore wish to apologize for any errors that may have slipped through during the editing process of this book.

With the introductory remarks out of the way, let's get started and examine the potential benefits strength training could bring you!

Why Seniors Should Work Out

I realize you are already aware that working out is beneficial to your health - otherwise, you wouldn't have bothered buying this book!

Don't worry, I am going to keep this section brief and to the point. Consider it a quick motivation boost before you get started or for whenever you don't feel like working out.

With that said, here is what regular strength training can do for you:

- Combating sarcopenia, the loss of muscle mass and strength as age increases
- Preserving bone density and thus lowering the risk of bone fractures
- Higher vitality
- Reducing risk, signs, and symptoms of many illnesses and chronic diseases, such as osteoporosis, heart disease, arthritis, type II diabetes, and depression
- Improving sleep
- Retaining independence and freedom
- Providing more resilience to injuries, like sprains and muscle tears
- Potentially alleviating joint and spine issues, including shoulder, neck, and back pain
- Making daily tasks much easier
- More balance and mobility, which could reduce the risk of falls
- Better posture
- Slightly improving cognitive function, memory, and mental health

In a nutshell, strength training may alleviate or prevent many common conditions older individuals face and thus helps preserve a good - if not great - quality of life.

In fact, a decently trained senior could very well maintain or reach the strength level of an average untrained person in their 30s. I understand, at first glance, you might think this is a little underwhelming - working out two to four times a week, just to get as strong as an *untrained* 30-year-old? Then again, if we look at it from a different angle, this doesn't seem bad at all.

Does an average 30-year-old person have any difficulties completing their daily tasks? Do they struggle walking upstairs, carrying their groceries, or playing with their kids? In the vast majority of cases, they don't.

Now, if I had to make an educated guess, I would say you don't want to work out (or start working out) to be able to deadlift 500 pounds or bench press twice your body weight. In all likelihood, you "just" want to improve or preserve your quality of life to continue to get by on your own indefinitely, without any issues or assistance.

And I daresay, in a society that offers only few physical challenges untrained people in their 30s cannot overcome, you may very well reach that goal.

This goes even if you have never picked up a weight before in your life. In fact, if you start lifting at 60, 70, or even 80 years old, the changes you will notice through weight training could be life-altering.

Sure, you cannot expect to gain as much muscle or strength as an average 20-year-old anymore. Then again, that doesn't matter. What matters is that you relieve or prevent pain as well as retain or regain your independence and freedom.

Workout Fundamentals for Seniors

To achieve this goal as effectively and efficiently as possible using the exercises in this book, it is important to keep a few basic training principles in mind. After all, it won't help you all that much if you just pick a few of these exercises but don't know how to apply them in a program.

That's why these principles answer a few basic questions, such as:

- Which exercise to pick for which body part?
- How much to train?
- How hard to train?
- How often to train?
- How to progress your training?
- And how to recover from training?

No worries, I try to avoid using complicated terminology and will keep this simple and easy to understand. Fortunately, resistance training is no rocket science and most of these guidelines are based in common sense, anyway.

First, let's go over these well-established and scientifically backed guidelines in a more general sense. This is how they apply for all people, regardless of gender or age.

Once we have covered this, we will examine how to adapt some of these principles to the needs and circumstances of seniors to make their training not only maximally effective but also maximally safe.

General Programming Basics

When talking about weight training, you will frequently encounter two basic terms - repetitions and sets. Let's briefly define these, in case you are not familiar with them:

- **Repetitions** (or reps for short) are the one-time complete execution of an exercise's range of motion. Squatting down from a standing position and then standing back up, for example, is one repetition of a squat.
- **Sets** are simply several consecutive repetitions without rest in between. Ten squats in a row, for example, are one set of ten squats.

When designing a routine to build muscle and strength, we must put these repetitions and sets in a larger context, though, by considering a few additional factors, which are:

Exercise selection

This means picking suitable exercises for each muscle group you wish to develop. A "good" exercise is safe to perform, causes its target muscle to be the limiting factor, and preferably causes little fatigue.

For example, the target muscle of a shoulder press is the front delt. If you can do this exercise pain-free and without joint discomfort, stop your sets because your shoulders get tired (and not your triceps or other supporting muscles), and the exercise doesn't cause pain or debilitating soreness afterwards, it is probably a "good" shoulder exercise.

Fortunately, you don't have to worry about this programming factor all that much because I provide you with lots of tried-and-tested exercises later!

Training volume

This refers to how much total work you do per week and workout for a certain muscle group. Usually, volume is simply the total number of working sets you do. Most beginners can already get great training results doing relatively low volume, starting at maybe 4-6 sets per muscle group per week. For intermediates with more training experience, I often give 8-12 weekly sets per muscle group as a guideline.

Relative effort

This principle means how close you get to true muscle failure in your working sets, or how hard you train. To get bigger and stronger muscles, we can't afford to go *too* easy on them, unfortunately. On the other hand, we also don't want to train them too intensely because this could lead to debilitating soreness, an increased risk of injury, and high mental fatigue.

Exercise science suggests that decent training results start to occur at about four or fewer so-called "repetitions in reserve". This means when you stop a set, you could have done a maximum of four more repetitions until muscle failure. The sweet spot probably lies around two reps in reserve for most muscle groups. That said, untrained people can get away with significantly easier training and still make great progress.

Repetition ranges

To build muscle and strength, you need to keep your working sets in a relevant repetition range. Science suggests any number of repetitions between 5 all the way up to 40 per set builds muscle about equally well, provided the set is taken close to failure. For optimal strength development and neurological adaptations, though, lower repetition ranges (fewer than 10 reps) are preferable.

Training frequency

Frequency answers the question how often to train a muscle per week. After all, you can't expect to make much progress if you only train once a month. Provided the weekly number of sets is the same, training a muscle once, twice, or three times a week seem to deliver similar results.

Progression

Progression is all about getting your muscles from point A (now) to point B (stronger than now). It entails to try to "get better" in your workouts over time, most commonly by adding weight, doing additional reps, or sometimes adding a set here and there.

Recovery

However, with all this training, recovery must also play an important role. Most muscles need around 24-72 hours of rest after a workout until you can train them effectively again, and joints and connective tissue need to recover as well.

Proper recovery management is vital to ensure consistency and progress in your training and to prevent injuries. This also encompasses your sleep and your nutrition.

Senior Specific Training Advice

Old age, unfortunately, entails some limitations when it comes to training, and building muscle and strength only gets harder and slower the older you get.

On top of that, seniors typically have a harder time recovering from joint stress and injuries. Muscle tears, sprains, or fractures could leave you bedridden for weeks and months or even end your training career altogether!

While someone younger may shrug off a small injury as if nothing happened, you may not have that luxury anymore. This means the number one guideline for seniors in their training is:

<u>Safety first.</u>

By extension, this means you cannot afford to be reckless when lifting weights. Going for one repetition maxes, pushing for additional repetitions while sacrificing technique, adding resistance when you have no business to… All this may lead to unnecessary and avoidable injuries.

Despite these challenges, seniors should still base their training on the above principles as well as they can. In most cases, they just need to be slightly adapted and individualized, preferably with the help of a physical therapist, doctor, or qualified personal trainer, in case you have specific limitations.

So, let's go through the programming basics again and examine some best practices for seniors.

Exercise selection

When seniors pick exercises, their choices should be aligned to their individual needs and abilities. For example, if you can't lift your arms overhead, you shouldn't program overhead presses but find other ways to stimulate your front and side delts. If you have bad hips, you should approach squatting and hip hinging exercises carefully and see which ones still work for you.

Weight training is highly individual, particularly for seniors who are more likely to have certain ailments and mobility limitations. Even though I am going to present you lots of different exercise options for each muscle group, it would be best practice to consult your doctor or physical therapist to check which of these are suitable for you if there is a joint that is giving you trouble.

Aside from personal abilities, you should also choose your exercises according to your training goals. For example, leg and back exercises probably have higher priority than biceps or chest exercises. Of course, you might still want to train "lower-priority" muscle groups to avoid imbalances. However, for most seniors and elderly people, strong legs and hips are more important than strong biceps and pecs.

Training volume

Too many intense working sets may cause severe muscle soreness if you are not accustomed to it yet. Same as someone younger, best start your training programs with conservative volume, like in the programs given at the end of this book.

For beginner seniors, this could mean as few as four working sets per muscle group per week.

Relative effort

Pushing sets too hard or even to failure can be dangerous for some seniors. Of course, it may still be an option and depend on the individual and which muscle group we are talking about. However, since failure training causes a lot more fatigue and joint stress at not much additional benefit compared to leaving a few repetitions in the tank, it is probably better to keep your intensity only reasonably hard. Take a set only to a point where it starts feeling tough, but you can still perform the exercise with perfect technique.

Repetition ranges

Lower repetition ranges mean that you must use heavier weights. Using heavier weights, though, means more joint stress and a (slightly) higher risk of injury. I am not saying lower repetition ranges are inherently dangerous and will cause you to get hurt. However, it is still a lot less likely to get injured doing sets of 10+ repetitions than it is doing sets of 5.

Remember, you want to be on the safest side when you train. That's why higher repetition ranges (10-30 repetitions per set) combined with reasonable relative effort are the way to go for the vast majority of your training.

Training frequency

Assuming sensible volume selection, there needn't be any changes on the training frequency front. Seniors should still try to hit all muscle groups one to three times per week.

Some people respond better to doing all their sets for a muscle group in one workout, while others prefer spreading out their working sets across several workout days. This may also be muscle group dependent.

For example, you may want to train biceps just once a week but hit back twice a week or train your hamstrings only once a week because they stay sore for so long.

At the end of the day, it won't matter much whether you do four sets of a muscle in one workout or two sets of a muscle in two workouts. As long as you are consistent with your training, both once-a-week-training and higher frequency training will deliver comparable results.

Progression

For younger people, progression should be the guiding principle in their training. For seniors, <u>safety</u> should be the guiding principle in their training. Even though you still try to increase your performance and work capacity over time, don't try to push for personal records if this means compromising safety. After all, you can't progress much anymore if you get injured.

It is okay to have a "bad" workout occasionally where you don't match your previous week's performance. What matters more is staying consistent with your training and free of injury. If you can do that, progression might even take care of itself.

Recovery

Recovery is a crucial training component for anyone, but for seniors it takes on an even more important role. Seniors often need notably longer to recover from joint stress and muscle soreness than younger people and are more prone to inflammation. That's why it is vital for you to rest adequately after your workouts - not just to reenergize yourself properly, but also to minimize injury risks and maximize safety.

And if this means taking one or two additional days off, then so be it.

To close this chapter, here are some training dos and don'ts for seniors, which summarize the above points.

Dos	Don'ts
Prioritizing safety	Prioritizing progression
Always maintaining proper form	Letting technique break down
Listening to your body	Pushing through discomfort or pain
Mainly going for higher repetition ranges	Going heavy too often
Prioritizing recovery	Training while overly sore
Relying on safe exercises and training principles	Doing potentially risky stunts
Leaving repetitions in the tank	Training to failure

77 Body Weight and Dumbbell Exercises for Seniors

Now that we have covered the theoretical basics, let's move on to the actual exercises and get practical!

This chapter begins with an overview of our body's different muscle groups to illustrate where they are and what they are called. We then work our way from top to bottom and examine each major muscle group in detail. I will give you a brief outline of its function, which priority it should take in your training, and of course which body weight and dumbbell exercises you can do to train it safely and effectively. Each exercise is given a difficulty level from 1 to 3, with 1's being particularly suitable for absolute beginners, 2's being a bit more technical, and 3's often requiring some existing strength foundation. Again, ability can vary greatly among seniors, which is why I wanted to include options for everyone. Regardless of your situation, I still highly recommend consulting your doctor to see which of these exercises are the best fit for you - especially if you have pre-existing conditions - and approaching each exercise carefully.

As for your dumbbells, an adjustable set from 5lbs to 30lbs or 40lbs per dumbbell would be best. Remember, the goal of any exercise is to get its target muscle reasonably close to failure anywhere between 10 to 30 repetitions. Make sure your dumbbells are heavy (or light) enough to stick to that guideline.

A few of these exercises require a training bench or incline bench. I included these because most of them are among the safest and lower-back-friendliest exercises out there. While there are many alternatives in case you don't have access to one, a stable and adjustable bench can still be a useful training tool for more exercise variety and lower back comfort.

However, that doesn't mean a bench or even a gym membership is a "must". After all, home training with dumbbells and body weight exercises alone can still get you very far and might be more than enough for your needs.

Each of the following exercises is accompanied by an illustration of start and end position, a description of how to perform it, and some notes and tips, in which I often present additional easier or harder variations to suit your level of ability.

If an exercise is new to you, best try the easiest variation of it for a couple of repetitions first and see how it feels to ensure maximum safety. For dumbbell exercises, this means either using your lightest set of dumbbells or performing the movement without weights altogether before jumping into a "real" set. As a matter of fact, warming up properly doing a few of these practice repetitions is general best practice for seniors.

Nevertheless, at the end of the day, I don't know you, which means I don't know which of these exercises are suitable for you personally, either. You might have a bad knee and must approach squatting very carefully. Your lower back could act up if you do exercises bent over. Or maybe you have shoulder problems and certain presses feel highly uncomfortable. This takes us back to our guiding principles from above:

When picking your exercises, listen to your body and prioritize safety.

If you're not sure or something feels off, please ask your doctor or physical therapist for guidance.

Anyway, enough with the introductory words. Now let's look at the muscles we want to strengthen and continue with the exercises!

Main Muscles of the Body - Front

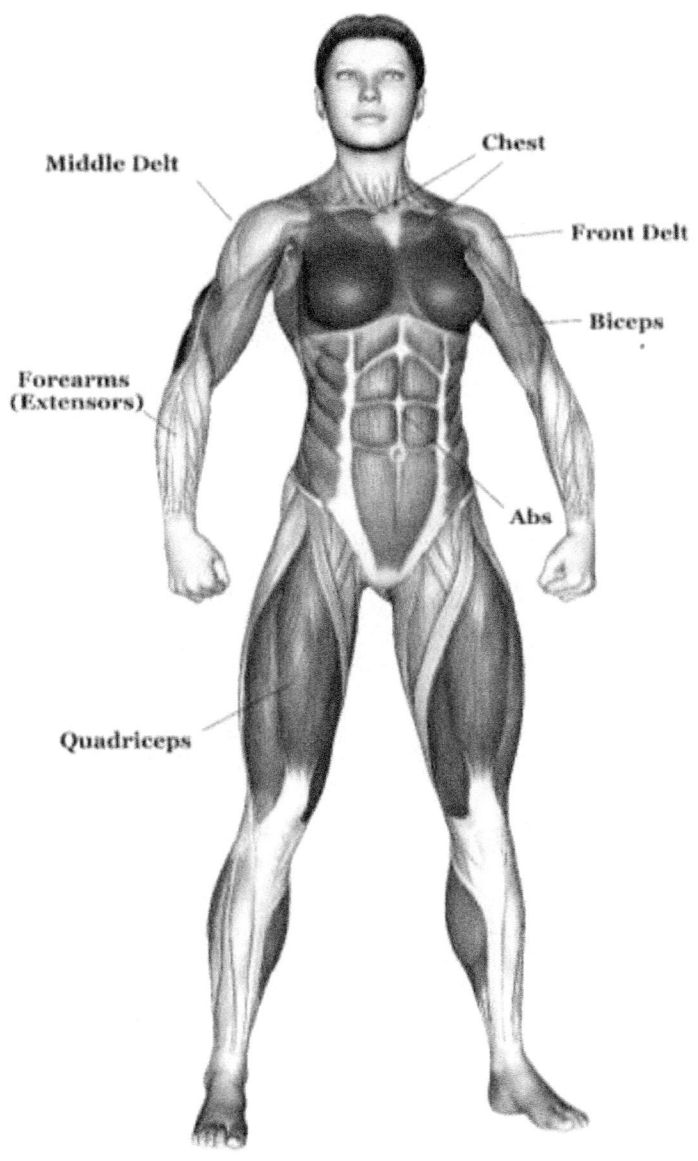

Main Muscles of the Body - Back

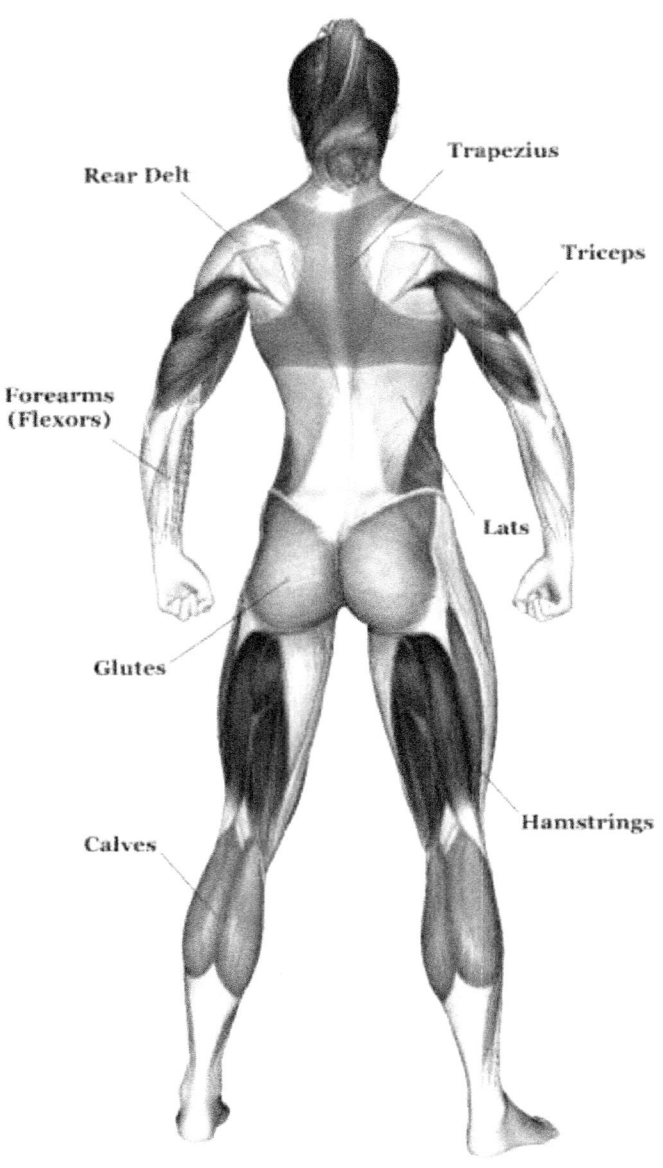

Shoulders

The shoulder consists of three distinct muscles, the front delts, the middle delts, and the rear delts. Each of these serve a different purpose and allow us to move our upper arms in all directions.

Since you need your shoulder muscles every time you move your arms, strengthening them can not only help you perform many daily tasks more easily (such as carrying objects in front of your body or performing tasks overhead), but also stabilize the joint and minimize the risk of injury.

How to work the shoulder:

- Front delts: Lifting the arm to the front and pushing objects overhead
- Middle delts: Lifting the arm to the side
- Rear delts: Lifting the arm to the back

Priority: moderate to high

Seated Dumbbell Shoulder Press

Difficulty: 1

Target muscle:
Front delts

Secondary muscle(s):
Triceps, side delts

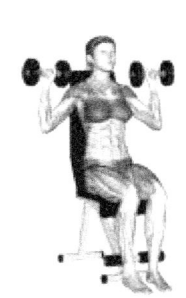
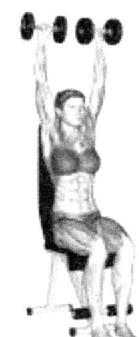

How to:

- Grab a pair of dumbbells and sit down on a chair or workout bench
- Palms facing forward, lift the dumbbells and rest them near your collar bones, so that your upper arms form a 30-45° angle with your torso
- Breathe in and engage your core, then push up the dumbbells directly above your head.
- Carefully lock out your elbows once you are all the way up, then slowly move the dumbbells back down until they touch the top of your shoulders.

Notes and tips:

Alternatively, you can do the dumbbell shoulder press while standing, using one arm at a time, or in a neutral grip, whichever is most comfortable for you.

In case you have mobility limitations and can't lift your arms overhead, though, best go with a front raise variation instead, which we will cover later.

Arnold Press

Difficulty: 1

Target muscle:
Front delts

Secondary muscle(s):
Triceps, side delts

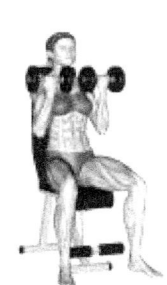 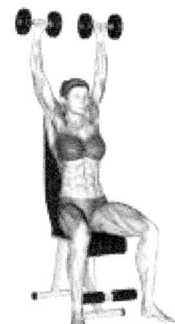

How to:

- Grab a pair of dumbbells and sit down on a chair or workout bench
- Hold the dumbbells at shoulder height, palms facing toward your face
- Press up the dumbbells, and as they go up, rotate your arms. In the top position, your palms face forward
- Reverse this motion on the way down - turn your palms towards you - until you reach the start position and repeat

Notes and tips:

This exercise was named after none other than Arnold Schwarzenegger himself and adds rotation to the standard dumbbell shoulder press. As such, it may also assist you on the shoulder mobility front.

Same as its rotation-free counterpart, you can do the Arnold press one arm at a time or standing.

Incline Dumbbell Shoulder Press

Difficulty: 1

Target muscle:
Front delts

Secondary muscle(s):
Triceps

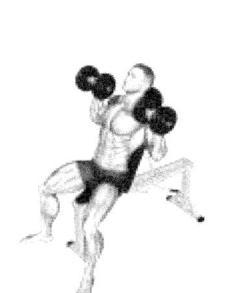 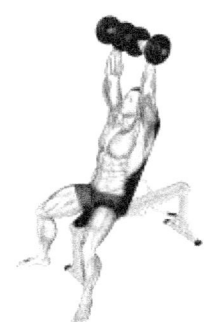

How to:

- Grab a pair of dumbbells and sit down on a relatively steep incline workout bench
- Hold your dumbbells at shoulder height, palms facing forward
- Breathe in and engage your core, then press the dumbbells straight up
- Reverse this motion on the way down as you breathe out. Make sure not to lose tension in your core.

Notes and tips:

Because of the incline angle at which you perform this shoulder press variation, it slightly favors the front part of your shoulder.

As with all other shoulder presses, it is perfectly fine to do the incline shoulder press one arm at a time or using a neutral grip.

Seated Front Raise

Difficulty: 1

Target muscle:
Front delts

Secondary muscle(s):
Side delts

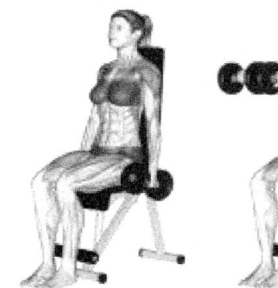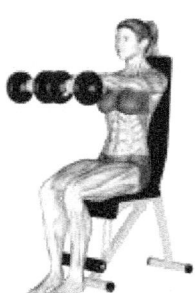

How to:

- Grab a pair of dumbbells and sit down on a chair or workout bench
- Hold the dumbbells next to your hips in a neutral grip
- Keeping your elbows straight, lift both dumbbells directly to the front until your arms are parallel to the floor (or however far you can get pain-free)
- You may maintain a neutral grip or rotate your arms inwards as you raise the dumbbells. When rotating your arms, though, best make sure your pinkie fingers don't go higher than your thumbs in the top position as this may cause shoulder discomfort
- Once you have reached the top position, slowly reverse the motion until you are back in the start position

Notes and tips:

Since some seniors may have issues raising their arms overhead, front raises could be a decent option to cover your front delts needs pain-free.

You can also do these standing, just be aware that this can be demanding on the lower back. To alleviate this, you may find it more comfortable to train one arm at a time.

Incline Front Raise

Difficulty: 1

Target muscle:
Front delts

Secondary muscle(s):
Side delts

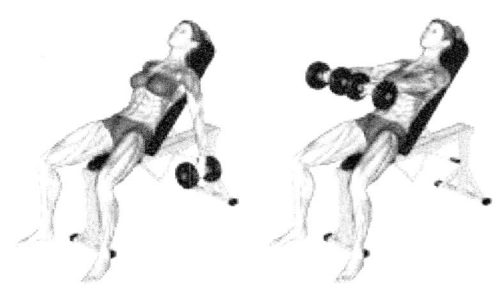

How to:

- Grab a pair of dumbbells and sit down on an incline bench
- Let the dumbbells hang down next to the bench and hold them in a neutral grip
- Keeping your elbows straight, lift both dumbbells directly to the front until your arms are parallel to the floor (or however far you can get pain-free)
- Again, feel free to maintain a neutral grip or rotate the dumbbells
- Once you have reached the top position, slowly reverse the motion until you are back in the start position

Notes and tips:

The incline angle offers a slightly different resistance curve, which means the exercise "feels harder" during a different portion of the lift - in this case, right after you start a repetition.

When building muscle and strength, it is usually a good idea to cover varying resistance curves for each muscle group to get stronger at various joint angles.

Seated Dumbbell Side Lateral Raise

Difficulty: 1

Target muscle: Side delts

Secondary muscle(s): Traps

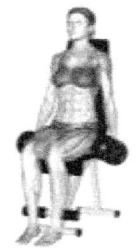 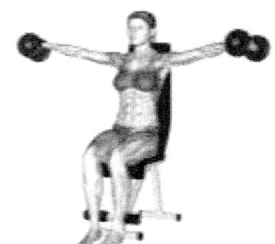

How to:

- Sit down on a chair or workout bench with a dumbbell in each hand
- Hold the dumbbells with your arms straight down at your sides
- Sitting as upright as possible and maintaining this position, lift both dumbbells to the side. Bend your elbows slightly and avoid swinging back and forth as you raise the dumbbells
- In the top position, when your arms are parallel to the floor, make sure your thumbs and pinkies are at the same height. Sometimes, it is recommended to "pour the pitchers", meaning tilting your hands forward, so your pinkies end up higher than your thumbs. However, this may cause shoulder discomfort.
- Reverse the motion until you are back in the start position

Notes and tips:

Aside from standing lateral raises, here are three worthwhile variations:

- **Bent-arm lateral raises**: Maintain a 90° bend in your elbows
- **Full-can lateral raises**: Lift the dumbbells with your thumbs turned all the way up. Note that this variation shifts the focus to the front delts.
- **Chest-supported lateral raises**: Sit down facing the back of a chair and lean into it as you do your lateral raises.

One Arm Lateral Raise with Support

Difficulty: 1

Target muscle: Side delts

Secondary muscle(s): Traps

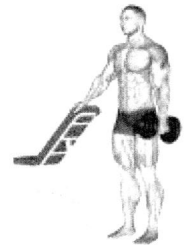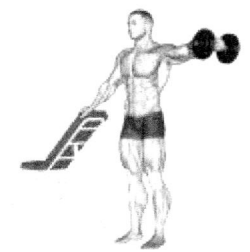

How to:

- Stand next to a training bench, chair, wall, other object to hold on to for stability and hold a dumbbell in one hand

- While supporting your balance with one hand, perform a dumbbell side lateral raise with the other. Keep in mind all the pointers of the two-handed variation

- Once you have completed your set, catch your breath for a second and proceed to train the other arm.

Notes and tips:

Unilateral training is particularly useful to detect and alleviate muscular imbalances, and it requires more stability work from your core.

If you are up for a more challenging version of this exercise with an altered resistance curve, you can try the leaning single arm dumbbell lateral raise. However, please note that this variation requires a lot more balancing and strength in your support arm and is only suitable for advanced folk!

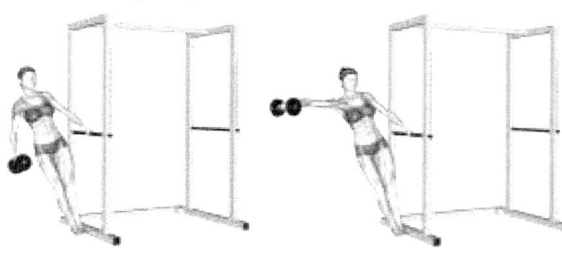

Hip Huggers

Difficulty: 1

Target muscle: Side delts

Secondary muscle(s):
Trapezius, rear delts

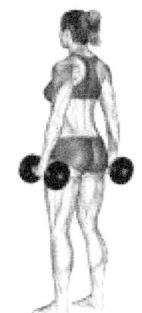 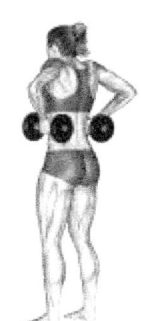

How to:

- Hold a pair of dumbbells at your sides while standing
- Make sure your core is stable and your back straight, then drag the dumbbells up your hips and waist
- Maintain a neutral grip and let your elbows travel backwards
- Hold the top position for a moment, then reverse the motion and repeat

Notes and tips:

This side delts exercise is a good option in case lateral raises cause pain or discomfort in your shoulders or wrists.

Of course, since the range of motion is much smaller and the focus arguably more on the rear delts, I would only pick hip huggers as main side delts exercise if your circumstances don't allow you to perform regular side lateral raises.

W-Press

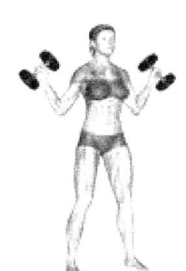 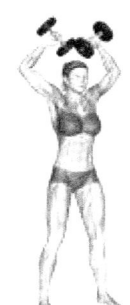

Difficulty: 2

Target muscle: Side delts

Secondary muscle(s):
Front delts

How to:

- While standing, hold a pair of dumbbells at head height with your arms to the sides and your elbows bent and tucked. From behind, your upper back area should look the letter "W"
- Maintaining a 90° angle in your elbows, push the dumbbells above your head until they touch. Make sure to engage your core to provide stability from below
- Reverse the motion until you are back in the start position and repeat

Notes and tips:

As almost all overhead presses, the W-Press also targets the front delts, making it a decent hybrid exercise for both front and side delts.

Naturally, you can perform this exercise also sitting down on a chair or workout bench.

Arm Circles

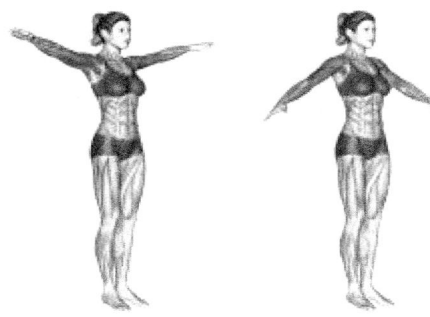

Difficulty: 1

Target muscle: Side delts

Secondary muscle(s): Front delts, rear delts

How to:

- While standing or sitting on a chair, hold your arms out to the side so that they are parallel to the floor
- Start rotating your arms forward by making small, controlled circular motions about 1 foot in diameter
- Go for about 20 to 30 seconds, then rest and repeat

Notes and tips:

Arm circles are more of an endurance exercise and particularly suitable for absolute beginners.

I mainly included these because they are an excellent way to warm up your shoulders and rotator cuff for your workouts.

That said, if you are looking for more of a challenge, you can consider doing arm circles holding a pair of dumbbells.

Bent Over Face Pull

Difficulty: 2

Target muscle: Rear delts

Secondary muscle(s): Upper back

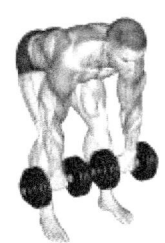 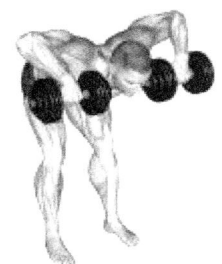

How to:

- Bend over from the hips while holding a pair of dumbbells and letting them hang straight down
- Make sure that your core is stable and your back straight
- Pull the dumbbells up towards your face by driving your elbows and shoulders behind your back
- To keep the focus on the rear shoulder, try to perform the exercise with relatively flared elbows
- Squeeze your shoulder blades at the top, then accompany the dumbbells back to the start position

Notes and tips:

If lower back issues prevent you from bending over pain-free, you can do this exercise either without bending over as much as shown in the illustration or while lying prone on an incline workout bench.

Seated Rear Delt Fly

Difficulty: 1

Target muscle: Rear delts

Secondary muscle(s): Upper back

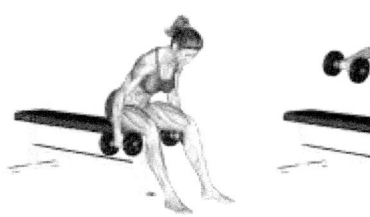

How to:

- Sit down on the edge of a workout bench or a chair
- Hold a pair of dumbbells next to your legs with straight arms and bend forward slightly
- Maintain stability in your core while lifting both dumbbells to the side with minimally bent arms
- Slowly reverse the motion until you are back in the start position

Notes and tips:

If your lower back allows it, it is also possible to do this exercise standing and bent over from the hip, like the above face pull.

Regardless of your chosen variation, be sure not to cheat with momentum and to get your elbows behind your back as far as your mobility allows it.

Incline Rear Delt Fly

Difficulty: 1

Target muscle: Rear delts

Secondary muscle(s): Upper back

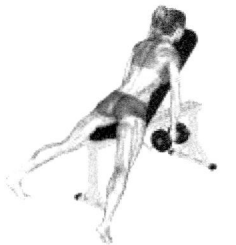 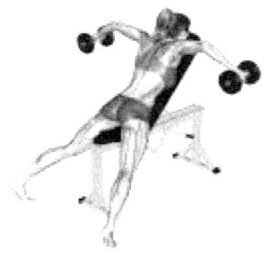

How to:

- Lie prone on an incline workout bench with a dumbbell in each hand, letting them hang straight down
- Same as with the regular rear delt fly, lift both dumbbells to the side until your elbows are behind your back and you feel a good squeeze in your upper back area
- Slowly reverse the motion until you are back in the start position

Notes and tips:

This version is particularly suitable for anyone struggling with lower back pain when bending over as the workout bench takes care of all the stabilization work.

Note that this exercise's incline angle also highly involves the upper back area.

Incline Y-Raise

Difficulty: 3

Target muscle: Upper back

Secondary muscle(s): Rear delts

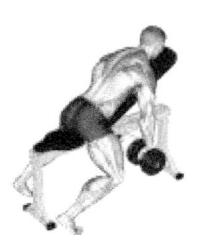
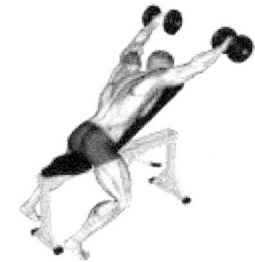

How to:

- Lie prone on an incline workout bench with a dumbbell in each hand, letting them hang straight down
- Lift the dumbbells to the front as high as you can
- Slowly reverse the motion until you are back in the start position

Notes and tips:

Not to be confused with the W-Press from earlier, the Y-Raise is an excellent exercise to strengthen the entire upper back area, including the rear delts.

Important to note here is that even the lightest dumbbells (or body weight only) can prove very challenging when doing this exercise, which is why it is probably better suited for more advanced seniors.

One Arm Reverse Fly with Support

Difficulty: 2

Target muscle: Rear delts

Secondary muscle(s): Upper back

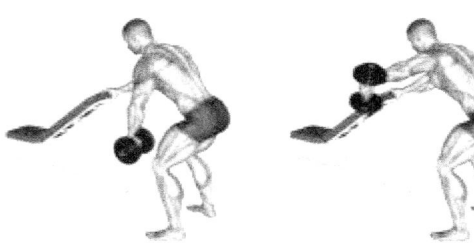

How to:

- Stand behind a workout bench or chair, holding on to the top end with one hand and carrying a dumbbell with the other. You can use a wall for support, too.
- While being bent over slightly, lift the dumbbell to the side, same as with a regular reverse fly
- Slowly reverse the motion until you are back in the start position
- Catch your breath for a few seconds and train the other arm once you feel ready

Notes and tips:

If your goal is to relieve strain off your lower back and you don't mind training each rear delt individually, consider this variation.

Some people may find it difficult to perform a rear fly with straight arms, though. In this case, it is also okay to keep your elbows bent while performing the exercise, even though, technically, this would be called a rear delt row.

However, the resulting training effect is similar, if not the same.

Back

A strong back is vital to protect the spine and complete everyday tasks, like carrying objects and picking things up from the floor. It also helps to alleviate postural problems and prevent pain in shoulders, neck, and spine.

The back consists of several interconnected muscles, which all serve similar functions. Chief among these are the trapezius, the rhomboids, the lats, and the spinal erectors of the lower back.

How to work the back:

- Pulling movements that have you move your arms behind your back. The higher you hold your elbows, the more you work the upper back. Lower elbow positions favor the lats.
- Straightening the torso from a bent over position, which mainly works the lower back and spinal erectors.

Priority: high

Bent Over Dumbbell Row

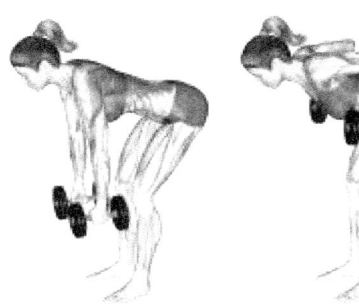

Difficulty: 2

Target muscle: Upper back

Secondary muscle(s):
Lats, rear delts

How to:

- Bend over from the hips while holding a pair of dumbbells and let them hang straight down. Try to "keep your chest up" as you bend over to prevent your lower back from rounding
- Maintain stability in your core and hold this position while pulling back the dumbbells next to your waist
- Keep your upper arms at a comfortable angle. Note that the more your flare out your elbows, the more you shift the exercise focus on the rear delts and traps.
- In the most contracted position, both your elbows and your shoulders should be as far back as possible.
- Make sure your back always straight during each stage of the exercise

Notes and tips:

Feel free to experiment with various wrist positions when doing this exercise and try it using a neutral grip or underhand grip. With the latter, you also indirectly involve the biceps, which can be a neat little benefit.

For more lower back comfort, try performing your rows leaning back into a wall while you are bent over. This should provide more support.

Bent Over Dumbbell Row with Chest Support

Difficulty: 1

Target muscle:
Upper back

Secondary muscle(s):
Lats, rear delts

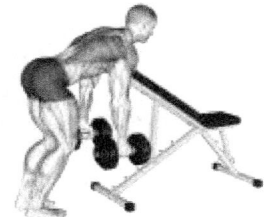 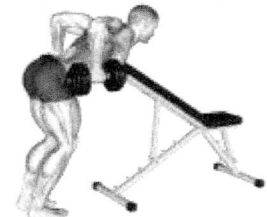

How to:

- Bend over from the hips while holding a pair of dumbbells and support your sternum on an incline bench or backrest of an armchair/sofa (but make sure your furniture can't slide away). Let the dumbbells hang straight down

- Maintain stability in your core while pulling back the dumbbells next to your waist

- Keep your upper arms at a comfortable angle. Note that the more your flare out your elbows, the more you shift the exercise focus on the rear delts and upper traps.

- In the most contracted position, both your elbows and your shoulders should be as far back as possible.

- Make sure your back always straight during each stage of the exercise

Notes and tips:

If lower back pain prevents you from doing bent over rows conventionally as described above, you can give this variation a try. Be sure not to place your chest too high as this might cause discomfort.

One-Arm Dumbbell Row

Difficulty: 2

Target muscle: Upper back

Secondary muscle(s):
Lats, rear delts

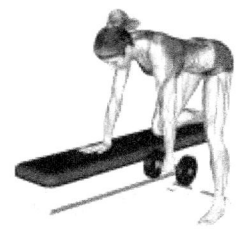 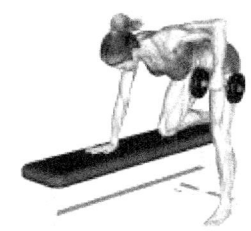

How to:

- Place your right hand and right lower leg on a workout bench (or something similar) while holding a dumbbell in your left hand and stabilizing with your left foot
- Maintain stability throughout your body and a straight back, then row the dumbbell next your waist area
- Drive your elbows and shoulders back behind your body but don't lose control or cheat too much with momentum
- Reverse the motion until you are back in the start position
- Complete a set for one arm, then switch to the other

Notes and tips:

As with most exercises, best experiment with different wrist positions - overhand, neutral, or underhand - and see which one works best for you.

Incline Dumbbell Row

Difficulty: 1

Target muscle: Upper back

Secondary muscle(s):
Lats, rear delt

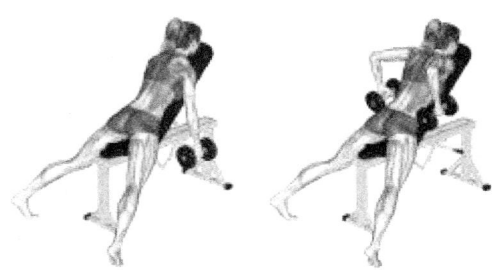

How to:

- Lie prone on an incline workout bench with a dumbbell in each hand, letting them hang straight down
- Same as with regular rowing variations, pull both dumbbells towards your waist while maintaining a comfortable upper arm/torso angle until your elbows are behind your back
- Slowly reverse the motion until you are back in the start position

Notes and tips:

The prone position and bench support of this rowing variation makes it a good option if you have lower back issues or suffer from vertigo if you bend over too far.

As always, using an underhand grip or neutral grip is perfectly okay.

Lying Prone Ws

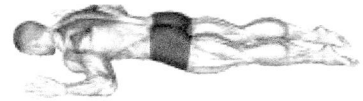

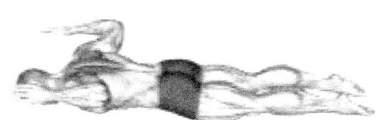

Difficulty: 2

Target muscle: Upper back

Secondary muscle(s): Rear delts

How to:

- Lie prone on an exercise mat with your arms spread out to the side and your elbows bent by 90°
- Breathe in, lift your elbows, and try to get them as high as possible
- Squeeze your shoulder blades in the top position and hold the tension for a moment
- Reverse the motion and get back in the start position as you breathe out

Notes and tips:

Like most movements performed in a prone position, this body weight upper back exercise is very easy on the lower back.

In case you have mobility issues in the shoulders, it is okay to cut the range of motion a bit. Raise your arms only as high as you can without pain.

Lying Prone As

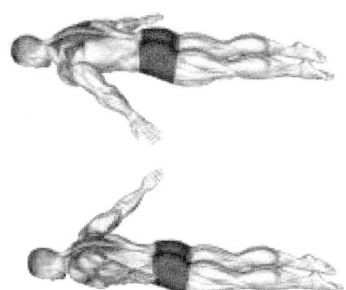

Difficulty: 2

Target muscle: Upper back

Secondary muscle(s): Rear delts

How to:

- Lie prone on an exercise mat with your arms spread out to the side and a 60° angle between your torso and upper arms
- Breathe in, lift your arms, and try to get them as far behind your back as possible
- Squeeze your shoulder blades in the top position and hold the tension for a moment
- Reverse the motion and get back in the start position as you breathe out

Notes and tips:

Compared to lying prone Ws, some people may find that lying prone As are easier on the shoulders and shift the focus on the mid back and lats.

Chest

For most seniors, strong pectorals won't rank high on the priority list. The chest is mainly responsible to bring the arm horizontally across the body, which is hardly ever needed in daily situations. That said, almost all pushing movements activate the chest, too, which is why movements involving the elbows and the shoulders may still have some carryover to everyday life.

For example, you may need your chest muscles to push open a heavy door or to push yourself up off the floor while lying on your stomach.

How to work the chest:

- Horizontal pushing movements.
- Horizontal adduction movements (i.e. bringing the arm across the body with resistance)

Priority: low to moderate

(Note: Even if a muscle group ranks low on the priority list, you should still include in in your training to avoid imbalances and to ensure overall strength)

Dumbbell Bench Press

Difficulty: 2

Target muscle: Chest

Secondary muscle(s): Front delts, triceps

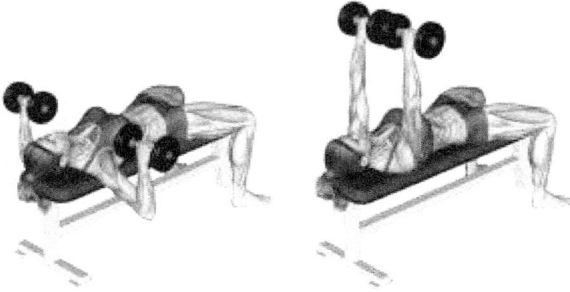

How to:

- Lie down on a flat workout bench with a dumbbell in each hand, placing them on the outside of your chest
- Keep your elbows at a comfortable angle between your torso - not too tucked and not too flared
- Pull your feet back and push your toes forward into the floor
- Create tension in your core, arch your back a bit, and squeeze your shoulder blades
- Breathe in and engage your core for stability, then push the dumbbells straight up
- Slowly lower the dumbbells back into the start position as you breathe out until they touch the outside of your chest

Notes and tips:

The dumbbell bench press is a time-tested and effective classic. In most cases, it is more shoulder-friendly than its barbell counterpart or push-ups because it allows you to move your arms freely in space. You can also do these using a neutral grip by turning your wrists 90° forward for potentially even more shoulder and wrist comfort.

Incline Dumbbell Bench Press

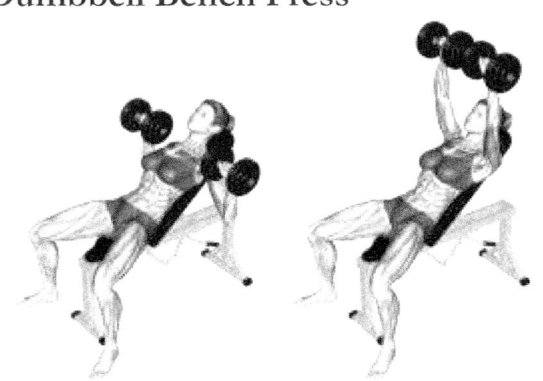

Difficulty: 2

Target muscle: Chest

Secondary muscle(s): Front delts, triceps

How to:

- Lie down on a 30° incline workout bench with a dumbbell in each hand, placing them on the outside of your chest
- Keep your elbows at a comfortable angle between your torso - not too tucked and not too flared
- Pull your feet back and push your toes forward into the floor
- Create tension in your core, arch your back, and squeeze your shoulder blades
- Breathe in and engage your core for stability, then push the dumbbells straight up
- Slowly lower the dumbbells back into the start position as you breathe out until they touch the outside of your chest

Notes and tips:

This exercise is a hybrid between a flat bench press and a shoulder press. As such, it will strengthen more of your upper chest and shoulder area than a conventional bench press. Also, some people find this variation gentler on the shoulders and easier to get into position.

Dumbbell Flys

Difficulty: 1

Target muscle: Chest

Secondary muscle(s): --

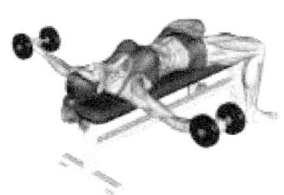 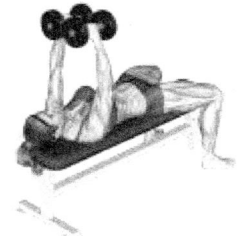

How to:

- Lie down on a flat workout bench and hold a pair of light dumbbells above your face with your palms facing each other
- Plant your feet firmly on the floor and make sure there is a slight bend at your elbows.
- Keeping this elbow position, lower the dumbbells to the side until you feel a decent stretch in your chest
- Reverse the motion until you are back in the start position

Notes and tips:

Dumbbell flys are a controversial exercise in the fitness community. Personally, I consider them rather safe, especially if you use light weights (or even no weights at all) and go for higher repetitions. As an added benefit, dumbbell flys help open the chest and improve scapular mobility, which could help reduce upper back pain and benefit your posture.

Naturally, you can also do dumbbell flys on an incline bench.

However, if you find this shoulder position uncomfortable or unstable, you can try our next two exercises as alternatives.

Hyght Dumbbell Flys

Difficulty: 1

Target muscle: Chest

Secondary muscle(s):
--

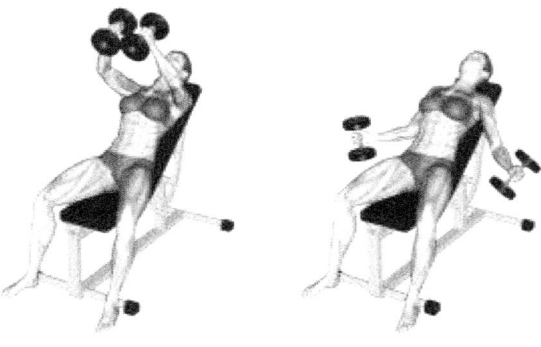

How to:

- Lie down on an incline workout bench and hold a pair of light dumbbells above your face with your palms facing each other
- Plant your feet firmly on the floor and make sure there is a slight bend at your elbows.
- Keeping this elbow position, lower the dumbbells to the side but at a more acute angle between torso and upper arms
- Reverse the motion until you are back in the start position

Notes and tips:

Because you keep your arms lower than with a regular dumbbell fly, many people find Hyght Fly much more comfortable in the shoulders.

You can also try these on a flat bench.

Floor Flys

Difficulty: 1

Target muscle: Chest

Secondary muscle(s): --

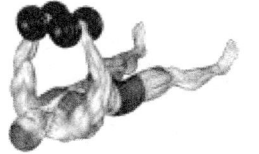 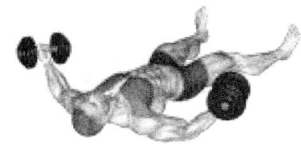

How to:

- Lie down on an exercise mat and hold a pair of light dumbbells above your face with your palms facing each other
- Make sure there is a slight bend at your elbows.
- Keeping this elbow position, lower the dumbbells to the side until your upper arms touch the floor
- Reverse the motion until you are back in the start position

Notes and tips:

Floor flys are the most beginner-friendly and safest fly exercise out there. Even though you sacrifice a little range of motion in the bottom position, this might be worth the additional "safety net" the floor provides.

For maximum shoulder comfort, try the Hyght floor fly, which uses a lower arm position.

Dumbbell Floor Press

Difficulty: 1

Target muscle: Chest

Secondary muscle(s): Front delts, triceps

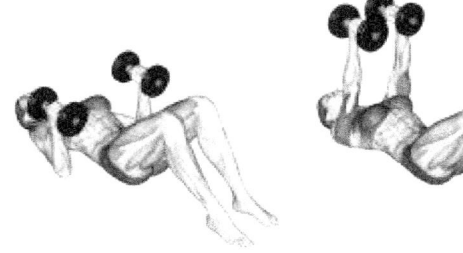

How to:

- Lie down on an exercise mat with your knees bent and rest your upper arms on the floor. Hold the dumbbells up with a 90° angle in your elbows.
- Push the dumbbells straight up while maintaining stability in your upper back
- Try to avoid flaring out your elbows too much for maximum safety and efficiency

Notes and tips:

The floor press may have the big drawback of not allowing as much range of motion than a regular dumbbell bench press. That said, if you prefer feeling maximally safe when doing your presses, it is still a valid option.

Some people may have issues getting both dumbbells into the start position due to wrist problems. In this case, best work out one arm at a time and assist your trained arm with your free hand to reach the proper start position without issues.

Push-ups

Difficulty: 3

Target muscle: Chest

Secondary muscle(s): Front delts, triceps

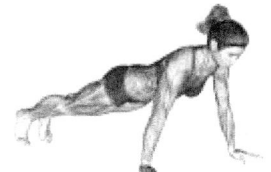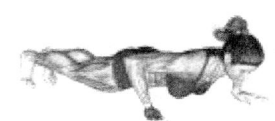

How to:

- Get down on all fours with your hands slightly further apart than shoulder width. Stretch out your legs and keep your feet about hip width apart, so you rest on your hands and toes.
- Tighten your core, glutes, and back to create stability throughout your mid-section
- Maintaining this tension, breathe in, bend your elbows, and lower yourself to the floor until your chest barely touches it
- Make sure your elbows don't flare out too much
- Push yourself back up into the start position

Notes and tips:

I realize that push-ups are probably a more advanced exercise for most seniors. Still, if you have the strength and mobility to do them properly and without pain, I highly recommend them. Not only are they very safe but they also build your chest, triceps, and shoulders effectively and strengthen a whole host of stabilizers throughout your mid-section.

For more wrist comfort, consider using push-up handles.

Kneeling Push-ups

Difficulty: 2

Target muscle: Chest

Secondary muscle(s):
Front delts, triceps

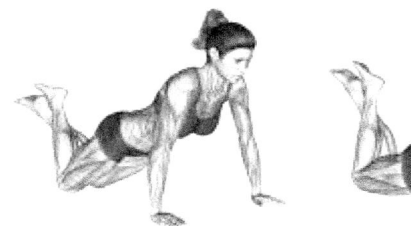

How to:

- Get down on all fours with your hands slightly further apart than shoulder width. Rest on your hands and lower legs
- Breathe in, bend your elbows, and lower yourself to the floor until your chest barely touches it
- Try to keep your chest up as you move down to prevent your upper back from rounding
- Make sure your elbows don't flare out too much
- Push yourself back up into the start position

Notes and tips:

If regular push-ups are (still) too hard for you, performing them on your knees is a great alternative.

For one thing, kneeling push-ups are easier on wrists and shoulders because need to you push less weight. For another, there is also less stabilization work required from your core, making it a highly beginner-friendly variation.

Incline Push-ups

Difficulty: 2

Target muscle: Chest

Secondary muscle(s): Front delts, triceps

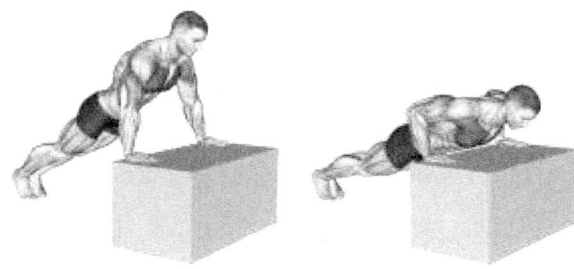

How to:

- Stand behind a table or similar stable elevated surface.
- Rest your hands on the edge and get into the start position of a push-up
- Create tension in your mid-section and glutes and lower yourself down while maintaining this tension
- Once your chest touches the elevated surface, push yourself back up into the start position.
- Make sure your legs and upper body form a straight line throughout each repetition

Notes and tips:

Incline push-ups are another good option for beginners to learn and master proper push-up form and develop their pushing muscles in the process.

I recommend starting with a relatively high surface (maybe 3-4 feet) and gradually choosing lower surfaces as you get stronger and more accustomed to the movement.

Wall Push-ups

Difficulty: 1

Target muscle: Chest

Secondary muscle(s): Front delts, triceps

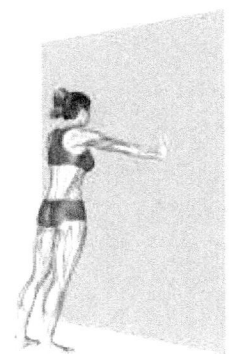 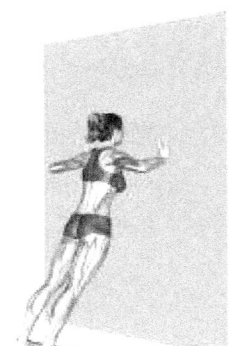

How to:

- Wear non-slip shoes, face a wall, and place your hands on it shoulder-width apart
- Stand about 2-3 feet away from the wall. The further away you stand, the more difficult the exercise becomes
- Create tension in your mid-section for stability
- Bend your elbows and lower your body towards the wall
- Once your head touches the wall, push yourself back to the start position.

Notes and tips:

Everyone has to start somewhere, and if the aforementioned push-up variations are all too difficult for you, maybe wall push-ups will do the trick.

If you have wrist issues, you could consider performing these while pressing a light set of dumbbells or push-up handles to the wall.

Biceps

The biceps are our primary elbow flexor and active, for example, when we carry an object in front of our chest with bent arms.

Many people see the biceps as more of a vanity muscle. While I agree that there are more important muscle groups to consider for seniors than the biceps, that doesn't mean you should ignore them in your training.

The biceps still play a supporting role in many daily activities, like picking things up from the floor or carrying grocery bags. Not to mention, stronger biceps may also help promote and protect elbow health.

How to work the biceps:

- Curling movements with the palms facing up
- Supination of the forearm (they "turn your pinkies up")

Priority: low

Dumbbell Biceps Curls

Difficulty: 1

Target muscle: Biceps

Secondary muscle(s): Forearms

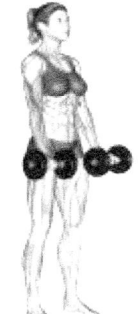 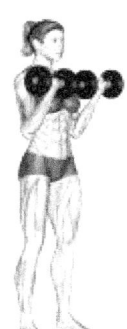

How to:

- While standing, hold a pair of dumbbells next to your waist with your palms facing forward and your pinkies turned up
- Create tension in your core to protect your lower back
- Maintaining this wrist position, keep your elbows tucked to your sides and curl up the weight
- Make sure your elbows stay tucked
- Slowly lower the dumbbells back into the start position

Notes and tips:

For more lower back comfort during curls, consider training one arm at a time.

Seated Biceps Curls

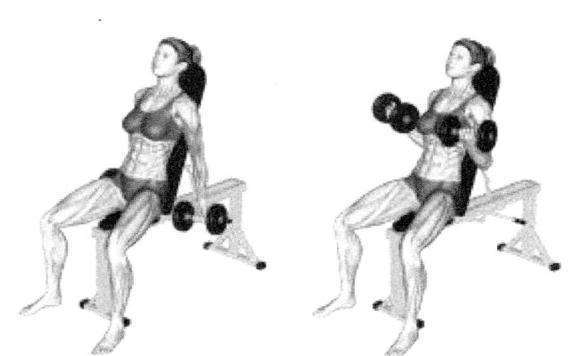

Difficulty: 1

Target muscle: Biceps

Secondary muscle(s): Forearms

How to:

- Sit down on a chair or workout bench and hold a pair of dumbbells next to your waist with your palms facing forward and your pinkies turned up
- Make sure your feet are firmly planted on the floor for stability
- Maintaining this wrist position, keep your elbows tucked to your sides and curl up the weight
- Slowly lower the dumbbells back into the start position

Notes and tips:

If your lower back acts up when doing your curls standing, consider seated biceps curls to help alleviate this issue.

Same as their standing counterpart, you can do these alternatingly as well.

Concentration Curls

Difficulty: 1

Target muscle: Biceps

Secondary muscle(s): Forearms

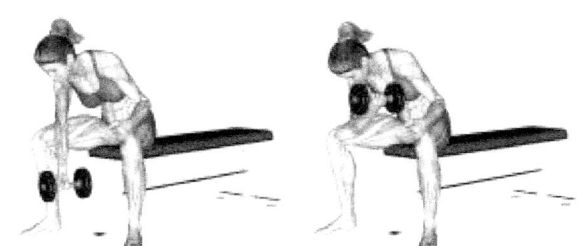

How to:

- Sit down on a workout bench while holding a dumbbell in your right hand.
- Slightly bend forward and place your right arm's elbow on the inside of your right leg's thigh, just above the knee
- Support yourself with your left hand by placing it on your left knee
- Keeping your elbow in position, curl up the weight
- Slowly reverse the motion until you are back in the start position

Notes and tips:

This one arm variation is a favorite among many lifters, both young and old. Since you are training one arm at a time, it allows you to fully focus on each biceps individually.

Concentration curls are also lower back friendly because you perform them seated.

Prone Incline Curls

Difficulty: 1

Target muscle: Biceps

Secondary muscle(s): Forearms

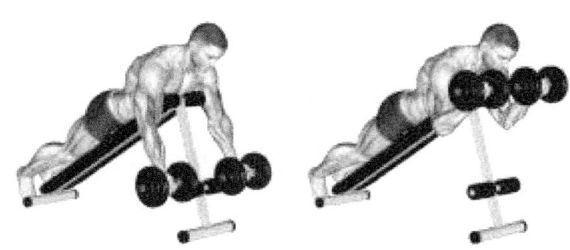

How to:

- Lie down on an incline bench in a prone position while holding a pair of dumbbells
- Palms facing forward, let the dumbbells hang straight down and turn up your pinkies
- Holding this wrist position, curl up the dumbbells without rocking your elbows forward
- Squeeze your biceps at the top, then reverse the motion until you are back in the start position

Notes and tips:

Prone incline curls, or spider curls, shift the curl's resistance curve to the end of the range of motion. As such, they are an ideal complement to regular curling variations performed standing or seated.

If your lower back allows it, you can also try these without the bench by curling while being bent over from the hips.

Triceps

As our main elbow extensor, the triceps are active during most pushing exercises for the shoulders and the chest. In everyday life, you may need your triceps when pushing yourself out of an armchair or from a lying position into a seated position.

Whether or not to include direct triceps work in your training is a highly individual question, though. If you are a beginner, chances are, you will work your triceps enough by focusing on your chest and shoulder presses alone.

That said, if you are more experienced or feel like your triceps need special attention, it can't hurt adding the odd triceps exercise here and there.

How to work the triceps:

- Extending the elbow during pressing and pushing movements

Priority: moderate

Close Grip Dumbbell Bench Press

Difficulty: 2

Target muscle: Triceps

Secondary muscle(s): Chest, front delts

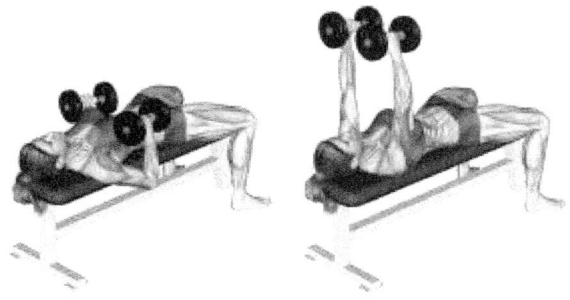

How to:

- Lie down on a flat workout bench with a dumbbell in each hand, placing them on the outside of your chest
- Keep your elbows tucked to your sides and hold the dumbbells in a neutral grip
- Pull your feet back and push your toes forward into the floor
- Create tension in your core, arch your back, and squeeze your shoulder blades
- Breathe in and engage your core for stability, then push the dumbbells straight up
- Slowly lower the dumbbells back to the start position as you breathe out until they touch the outside of your chest

Notes and tips:

The only difference between this bench press variation and the regular dumbbell bench press is the arm/torso angle. By keeping your elbows tucked, the chest muscles can't assist the movement as effectively - which means the triceps must do more work.

If you train without a bench, you can do these on the floor, too.

Dumbbell Triceps Extensions

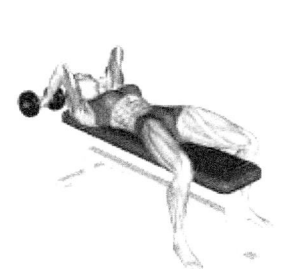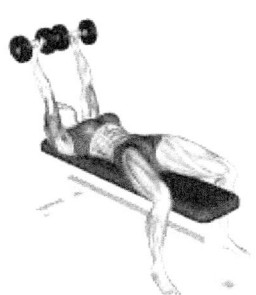

Difficulty: 2

Target muscle:
Triceps

Secondary muscle(s):
--

How to:

- Lie down on a flat workout bench, holding a pair of dumbbells above your head. Your arms are straight, and your palms face forward
- Tilt your arms slightly back, and plant your feet firmly on the floor
- Maintaining this shoulder angle throughout your set, lower the dumbbells behind your head by bending your elbows
- Once you are all the way down, reverse the motion until you are back in the start position

Notes and tips:

In case you don't have access to a training bench, it is also perfectly fine to do this exercise lying on the floor. This even makes it a little safer because the floor can act as your "safety net" again.

Some people find this exercise a bit tough on the elbows, though. Best start with light to moderate weights, and if this doesn't help, consider our next exercise.

Incline Dumbbell Triceps Extensions

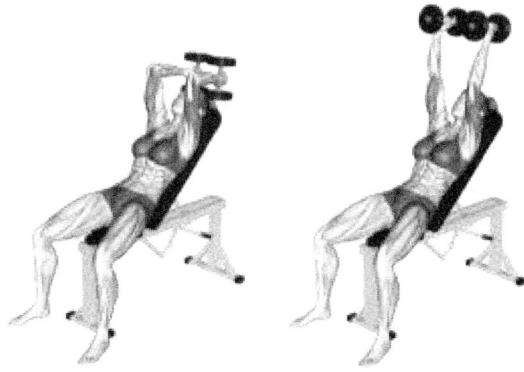

Difficulty: 2

Target muscle: Triceps

Secondary muscle(s):
--

How to:

- Sit down on an incline workout bench, holding a pair of dumbbells above your head. Your arms are straight, and your palms face each other

- Tilt your arms slightly back, and plant your feet firmly on the floor

- Maintaining this shoulder angle throughout your set, lower the dumbbells behind your head by bending your elbows

- Once you are all the way down, reverse the motion until you are back in the start position

Notes and tips:

As I mentioned above, this variation's incline angle shifts some strain away from the elbows, making it the go-to alternative for beginners or seniors with elbow issues.

Incline Dumbbell French Press

Difficulty: 2

Target muscle: Triceps

Secondary muscle(s):
--

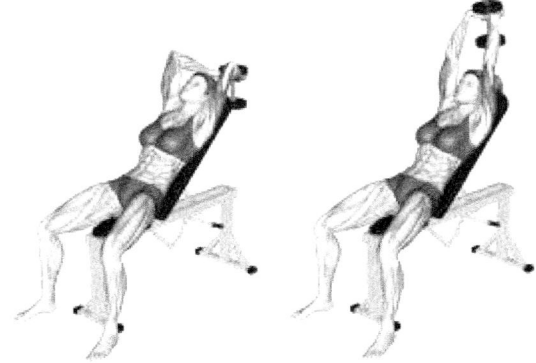

How to:

- Sit down on an incline workout bench
- Grab a dumbbell by the weight plate with both hands and raise it above your head
- Keeping your shoulders fixed in position, slowly lower the dumbbell behind your head by bending your elbows
- Make sure to avoid flaring out your elbows too much
- Push the dumbbell back up using the strength of your triceps

Notes and tips:

The incline French press is a great option if you prefer more stability during your triceps extensions.

You can do this exercise also while standing or seated on a chair or flat bench. However, doing French presses more vertically is slightly tougher on the elbows and shoulders.

Close Grip Push-ups on Knees

Difficulty: 2

Target muscle: Triceps

Secondary muscle(s): Chest, front delts

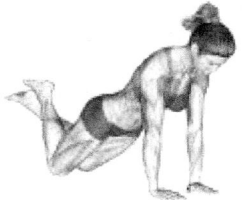 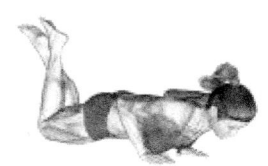

How to:

- Get down on all fours with your hands shoulder width apart. Rest on your hands and knees
- Breathe in, bend your elbows, and lower yourself to the floor until your chest barely touches it. Keep your elbows tucked
- Try to keep your chest up as you move down to prevent your upper back from rounding
- Push yourself back up to the start position

Notes and tips:

Same as the close grip dumbbell bench press, close grip push-ups reduce the involvement of the chest in the movement.

As with all push-up variations, consider using push-up handles if you have wrist issues.

Cobra Push-ups on Knees

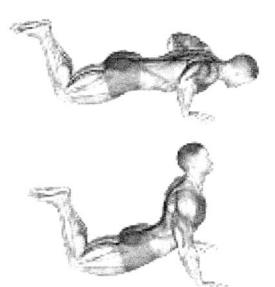

Difficulty: 3

Target muscle: Triceps

Secondary muscle(s): Chest, front delts

How to:

- Get down on all fours with your hands shoulder width apart. Rest on your hands and knees.
- Breathe in, bend your elbows, and lower yourself to the bottom position of a kneeling push-up. Keep your elbows tucked
- Try to keep your chest up as you move down to prevent your upper back from rounding
- As you push yourself back up, extend your back and fully contract your triceps.
- Get back into the bottom position and repeat

Notes and tips:

Cobra push-ups have you move your arms behind your back as you push yourself up, which hast the triceps do even more work.

As such, this variation is probably more suitable for advanced seniors.

Wall Pulse

Difficulty: 1

Target muscle: Triceps

Secondary muscle(s):
--

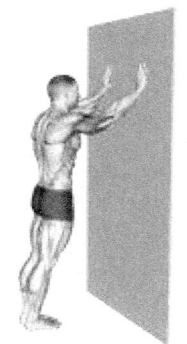 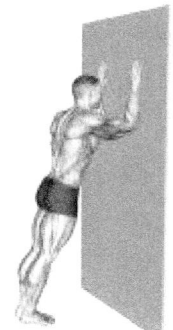

How to:

- Wear non-slip shoes, face a wall, and place your hands on it about shoulder-width apart and slightly above head height

- Stand about 2-3 feet away from the wall. The further away you stand, the more difficult the exercise becomes

- Create tension in your mid-section for stability

- Bend your elbows without flaring them out and lower your body towards the wall

- Once your head touches the wall, push yourself back into the start position.

Notes and tips:

Wall pulses are a particularly beginner- and joint-friendly triceps exercise.

You may want to experiment with a few different hand placements (maybe a bit higher, maybe a bit lower) to see which one works best for you.

Forearms

The forearms consist of wrist extensors and wrist flexors and are responsible for our grip strength and moving the wrist and fingers.

Whenever you firmly hold on to a railing or carry something with a closed fist, you need your forearms, which makes them an important muscle for seniors.

Many exercises work the forearms isometrically by having to maintain a firm grip on the dumbbells, which has a lot of carry-over to everyday life in and of itself.

Still, some direct forearm training can't hurt to put the cherry on the cake.

How to work the triceps:

- Curling movements with the palms facing forwards (flexors)
- Curling movements with the palms facing backwards (extensors)

Priority: moderate

Reverse Curls

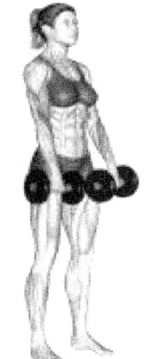 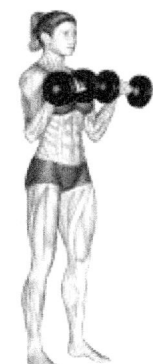

Difficulty: 1

Target muscle:
Forearm extensors

Secondary muscle(s):
Biceps

How to:

- While standing, hold a pair of dumbbells next to your waist with your palms facing backwards
- Create tension in your core to protect your lower back
- Keep your elbows tucked to your sides and curl up the weight
- Slowly lower the dumbbells back into the start position

Notes and tips:

Movement-wise, this exercise closely resembles a biceps curl, the only difference being that you use an overhand grip with this one.

This pronated grip takes the biceps mostly out of the equation and has the forearm extensors, chiefly among them the *brachioradialis*, and the *brachialis*, our secondary elbow flexor, do more work.

As with most curl variations, feel free to either train both arms at a time or each arm individually, whichever you prefer.

Behind the Back Finger Curls

Difficulty: 1

Target muscle:
Forearm flexors

Secondary muscle(s):
--

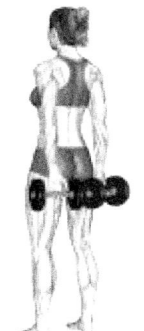 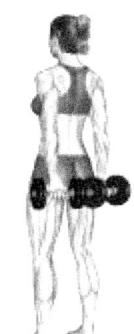

How to:

- While standing, hold a pair of dumbbells behind your back with hanging arms
- Keeping your arms in position, curl up the weights with your wrists with your palms facing away from your body
- Hold the maximum tension for a moment, then reverse the motion and repeat

Notes and tips:

Initially, I was reluctant to include a forearm flexor exercise because these may be tough on the wrists for some people.

However, you may not be "some people".

Since wrist curls are still a good exercise to improve grip strength, I recommend giving these a shot and see how your wrists tolerate them.

Cross-Body Hammer Curls

Difficulty: 2

Target muscle: Brachialis

Secondary muscle(s):
Forearm extensors, Biceps

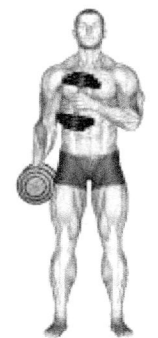
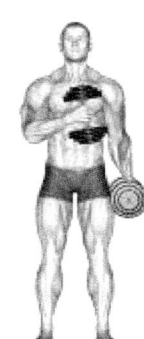

How to:

- While standing, hold a pair of dumbbells slightly in front of your waist in a neutral grip
- Create tension in your core to protect your lower back
- Keeping your elbows fixed to your sides, curl up one dumbbell at a time across your body
- Slowly lower the dumbbell back into the start position
- Switch sides after each repetition

Notes and tips:

The cross-body hammer curl isn't a pure forearm exercise as it also involves the brachialis and to lesser extent the biceps, which are both upper arm muscles.

Still, it is just too good an exercise for us to ignore, and since I didn't include a "hybrid" category, I figured now is a good a time as any to mention them.

Farmer's Carry

Difficulty: 2

Target muscle:
Forearms

Secondary muscle(s):
Quads, upper back

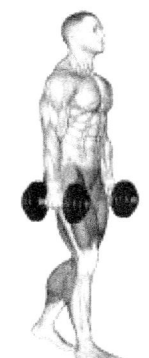 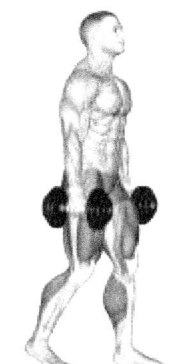

How to:

- While standing, hold a reasonably heavy pair of dumbbells at your sides
- Keep your shoulders back and an upright posture and create tension in your core to protect your lower back
- Start walking while maintaining good shoulder and upper back posture

Notes and tips:

The farmer's carry may easily be one of the best exercises to develop isometric strength in your forearms and upper back. It is also highly functional and has a lot of carry-over (pun intended) to the real world.

Think carrying grocery bags, water jugs, suitcases, gardening tools (like shovels) and other objects from point A to point B. This exercise will not only help you improve your grip strength for these tasks but also develop your cardiovascular endurance and balance. Just make sure you have a clear walking path without any tripping hazards. Beginners may also perform this exercise just shifting their weight from foot to foot instead of walking around.

Suitcase Carry

Difficulty: 3

Target muscle:
Forearms

Secondary muscle(s):
Quads, upper back

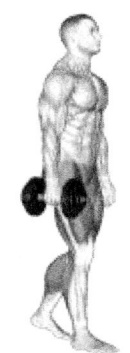 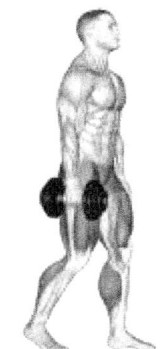

How to:

- While standing, hold one reasonably heavy dumbbell at your side
- Keep your shoulders back, maintain an upright posture, and create tension in your core to protect your lower back
- Start walking while maintaining good shoulder and upper back posture
- Be mindful not to lean towards your loaded side. Actively work against it by keeping your opposite obliques engaged.

Notes and tips:

Even though the suitcase carry is closely related to the farmer's carry, I figured it warrants its own entry in this book. After all, you are far more likely to carry something in just one hand than two items of equal weight at the same time.

Since you are "loaded" only on one side, though, there is a lot more stabilization work required, both from your legs and your core.

That's why this exercise is probably only suitable for more robust seniors or with conservative weight selection.

Abs

Some younger people primarily work out for aesthetics, and having visible abs is one of their main reasons to do strength training.

As a senior, you probably don't care about that anymore. Still, strong abs can help protect the spine and internal organs when you pick up objects from the floor as well as support good posture and even assist with breathing. As such, a few direct abs exercises should find their way into your program.

How to work the abs:

- Rounding the spine, either by bringing the rib cage close to a fixed pelvis (as during a crunch) or by bringing the pelvis close to a fixed rib cage (as during a leg raise)
- Adding rotation to these movements will also involve the obliques

Priority: moderate

Long Arm Crunch

Difficulty: 2

Target muscle:
Upper abs

Secondary muscle(s):
--

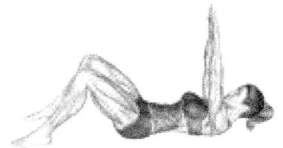 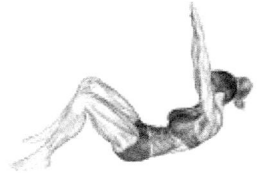

How to:

- Lie down on an exercise mat with your knees bent and extend your arms upwards
- From this position, lift your chest area off the floor by engaging your abdominals
- Actively try to round your upper back, then move back into the start position.

Notes and tips:

Traditional sit-ups can be tough on the lower back, particularly if someone has a preexisting condition.

Fortunately, you can train your abs without taxing your lower back all that much if you choose this crunch variation.

To make this exercise more challenging, consider holding a dumbbell as you do it. Beginners may rest their arms on their chest.

Quarter Sit-ups

Difficulty: 1

Target muscle:
Upper abs

Secondary muscle(s): --

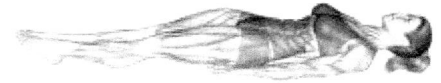
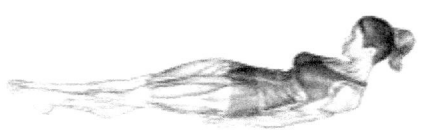

How to:

- Lie down on an exercise mat with your legs stretched out.
- Keep your arms next to your sides
- From this position, lift your chest area off the floor by engaging your abdominals
- Actively try to round your upper back, then move back into the start position.

Notes and tips:

In case long arm crunches are a tad too challenging for you, consider quarter sit-ups. These are also lower back friendly and a good option to strengthen the upper abdominals.

In the bottom position, you have two options:

- Disengage your abs for a moment before starting your next repetition by briefly lying down
- Maintain the tension by not resting on the floor

Best choose whichever option allows you to reach 10+ repetitions.

Spell Caster

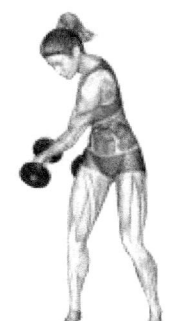 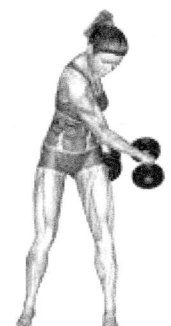

Difficulty: 2

Target muscle:
Obliques

Secondary muscle(s):
--

How to:

- Hold a pair of dumbbells in an overhand grip and assume a stable stance
- Move both dumbbells to one side next to your hip, rotating your torso.
- Rotate your torso to move the dumbbells to the other side, while keeping your arms straight. Make sure to perform this motion carefully and under control
- Continue switching from side to side until your set is complete

Notes and tips:

If you are a beginner, you might want to do this exercise with very light dumbbells or using bodyweight only for the time being, just to get a feel for it.

Spinal rotation can be tricky for the lower back if you are not careful, so be sure not to lose control or use momentum.

Twisting Crunch

Difficulty: 2

Target muscle:
Obliques

Secondary muscle(s):
Upper abs

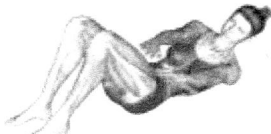 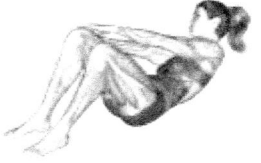

How to:

- Lie down on an exercise mat with your knees bent and extend your arms forwards
- From this position, lift your chest area off the floor by engaging your abdominals and slightly twist to the left
- In the maximum contracted position, both arms are to the right of the knees
- Move back to the start position, then do a crunch to the left

Notes and tips:

If you prefer more stability and less lower back involvement when training your obliques, try the twisting crunch.

To make this exercise more challenging, you can also do it while holding a dumbbell in both hands

Bottoms Up

Difficulty: 1

Target muscle:
Lower abs

Secondary muscle(s):
Hip flexors

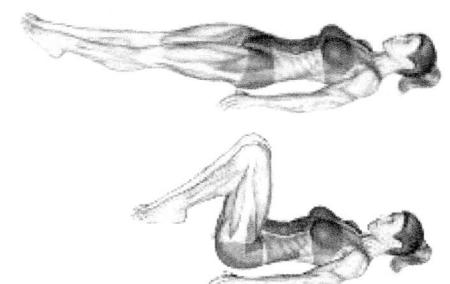

How to:

- Lie down on an exercise mat with your legs stretched out.
- Keep your arms next to your sides to stabilize yourself
- Pull your knees towards your chest and bend your legs on the way up
- Lift your bottom slightly off the floor in the maximum contracted position, then move back to the start position

Notes and tips:

Beginners may want to rest their legs briefly on the floor after each repetition. If you are more advanced, keep your legs in the air throughout your set to maintain tension in your abs and legs.

Hip Lift

Difficulty: 3

Target muscle:
Lower abs

Secondary muscle(s):
Triceps

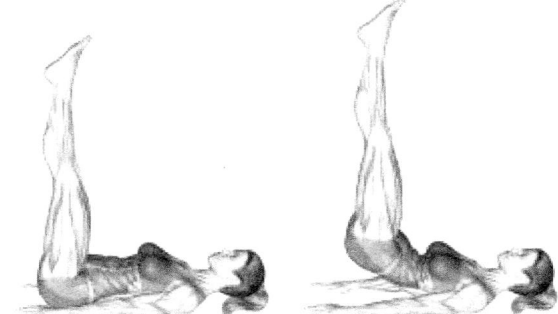

How to:

- Lie down on an exercise mat with the soles of your feet pointing to the ceiling
- Keep your arms next to your sides to stabilize yourself
- Lift your pelvis off the ground by engaging your abs - try to "touch the ceiling" with your feet
- As you push up your legs, push your arms down for support
- Reverse the motion to get back into the start position

Notes and tips:

Funnily enough, this exercise can also get quite challenging for the triceps as you keep stabilizing with your arms.

Speaking of stability, try to avoid swinging too much back and forth with your legs. They should move up and down in a straight line.

Kneeling Plank

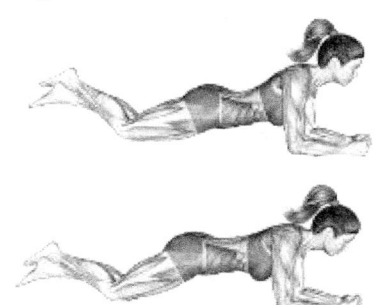

Difficulty: 1

Target muscle:
Abs

Secondary muscle(s):
Quads

How to:

- Get down on all fours with your arms shoulder width apart. Rest on your forearms and thighs
- Breathe in and lift your thighs off the floor. Make sure your back remains straight
- Hold this position by engaging your abs

Notes and tips:

This is the easiest plank variation, which might be a good starting point for some seniors. Its isometric contraction assists in developing the stabilizing function of the abs, which is crucial to protect the spine.

If you are looking for more of a challenge, though, perform the regular version of the exercise by resting on your toes instead of your knees.

Forward Step Front Plank

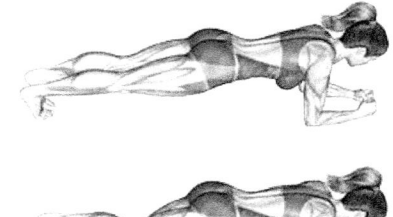

Difficulty: 2

Target muscle:
Abs

Secondary muscle(s):
Quads, shoulders

How to:

- Get down on all fours with your arms shoulder width apart. Rest on your forearms and toes and make sure your back and legs form a straight line
- Hold this position by engaging your abs
- Alternatingly move your left and right forearms a few inches forwards and pull them back again
- Repeat for the duration of your set

Notes and tips:

More advanced plank variations add movement to the exercise. This is just one of many different options, and I encourage you to get creative with your planks to keep them challenging. For example:

- Lift your legs alternatingly
- Move your forearms to the side
- Lift one arm to the front
- Move one knee towards your elbow

Quads

…or quadriceps for long. Our first group of leg muscles on the agenda is easily one of the most important muscle groups for any senior.

As main knee extensor, the quads are active when we walk, run, jump, and squat. Every time you take the stairs or get up out of a chair, you need this muscle. If the quads are strong, you may also improve your balance and protect your knee joint, thus reduce the risk of injury in that area and more easily prevent falls.

Regardless of your situation, try to find a few exercises to get this muscle as strong as you can for maximum quality of life.

How to work the quads:

- Getting up from a kneeling or squatting position by extending the knee joint

Priority: high

Body Weight Squat

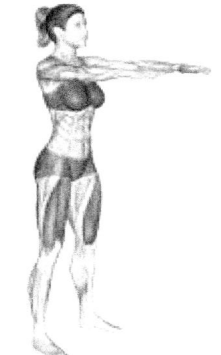
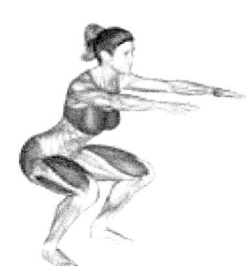

Difficulty: 2

Target muscle:
Quads

Secondary muscle(s):
Glutes, lower back

How to:

- Assume a comfortable stance width for squatting. For most people, this is somewhere around hip to shoulder width. Your toes may point slightly outwards or directly forwards, whichever feels more natural to you

- Tighten your core, inhale, and sit down into the squat with your arms stretched out in front of you for balance. Try to keep your chest up, your back straight, and your low bearing joints aligned

- As you descend, your hips move backwards and your knees travel forwards. Pretend you are sitting down on an imaginary chair - this may help you maintain proper form

- In the bottom position, your thighs should be parallel to the ground and your feet firmly planted on the floor

- Maintain an upright posture and stand back up to reach the start position. Push from your mid-foot to engage both quadriceps and glutes.

Notes and tips:

Squats are one of the more technical movements, so here are a few pointers to help prevent discomfort and ensure safe training results:

- **Don't let your knees cave in.** Try to maintain proper joint alignment by keeping your hips stacked over your heels and your knees stacked over your ankles.
- **Squat only as deep as you comfortably can.** Don't force yourself to reach squat depth if you still lack the mobility for it. A squat slightly higher than parallel is also okay.
- **Don't lift your heels off the ground.** This might cause excessive knee travel and cause discomfort. Adapt your stance or put a small object (like a dumbbell weight plate) under your heels while you squat to alleviate this issue.
- **Reach "true depth".** Some people heavily bend forward from the hips as they squat, which makes the movement very hip dominant. To keep the focus on the quads, best train in front of a mirror to check your knee angle and whether your thighs actually get (close to) parallel to the floor.
- **Focus on your core.** Don't forget to maintain the tension in your core to stabilize your spine and protect your lower back. Contract your abs before you squat down and inhale into this tension. Exhale as you stand up, then reset once you are fully erect.
- **(Optionally) Hold on to something stable** for added stability, like the backrest of a chair or sofa. Make sure this object can't slide away, though.

Dumbbell Bench Squat

Difficulty: 1

Target muscle:
Quads

Secondary muscle(s):
Glutes, lower back

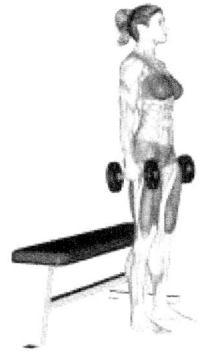 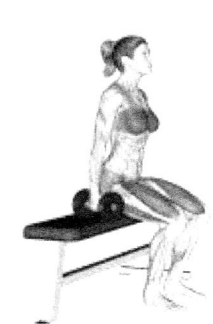

How to:

- Stand in front of a workout bench or chair while holding a pair of dumbbells at your sides
- Assume a comfortable stance width
- Tighten your core, inhale, and sit down. Try to keep your chest up and your back straight
- Stand back up while maintaining an upright posture
- Rest for a second, then go for the next repetition

Notes and tips:

This is the most beginner-friendly squat variation, which could be the ideal first quads exercise for some seniors. Here is how you can adapt it further to your fitness level:

- To make it easier, train without dumbbells and/or choose a higher chair
- To make it harder, use heavier dumbbells, choose a lower chair, and/or do not rest your buttocks on the bench between repetitions

Goblet Squat

Difficulty: 2

Target muscle:
Quads

Secondary muscle(s):
Glutes, lower back

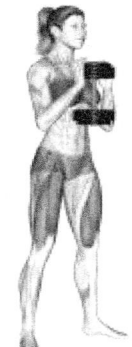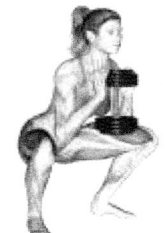

How to:

- Assume a comfortable stance for squatting and hold a dumbbell in both hands

- Tighten your core, inhale, and go down into the squat. Make sure to keep in mind all pointers of a regular body weight squat, which I outlined above

- Maintain an upright posture and stand up into the start position

Notes and tips:

Goblet squats are another beginner-friendly squat variation. You may find that holding a dumbbell in front of your body makes it easier to maintain an upright posture and keep your heels on the floor.

If you are having difficulties holding the dumbbell like in the above illustration, you can also let your arms hang straight down.

Dumbbell Wall Squat with Stability Ball

Difficulty: 2

Target muscle:
Quads

Secondary muscle(s):
Glutes, lower back

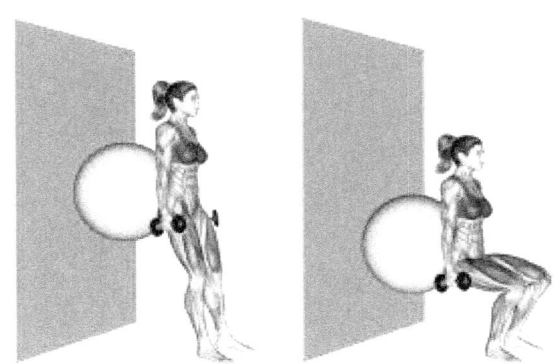

How to:

- Place a stability ball between a wall and your lower back

- Assume a comfortable stance for squatting while holding a pair of dumbbells and lean back into the ball

- Tighten your core, inhale, and go down into the squat. Make sure to keep in mind all pointers of a regular body weight squat, which I outlined above

- Maintain an upright posture and stand back up

Notes and tips:

I realize this squat variation requires an additional piece of equipment; however, it is just too good an option for some seniors to be left out of this book.

Wall squats with a stability ball make it a lot easier to maintain an upright posture and take care of most of the stability work. This may allow you to work your quads more effectively.

For added safety, consider placing a low stool underneath your buttocks.

Dumbbell Squat

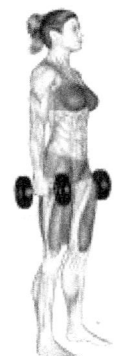 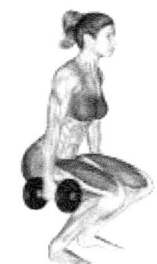

Difficulty: 2

Target muscle:
Quads

Secondary muscle(s):
Glutes, lower back

How to:

- Assume a comfortable stance for squatting while holding a pair of dumbbells at your sides

- Tighten your core, inhale, and go down into the squat. Make sure to keep in mind all pointers of a regular body weight squat, which I outlined above

- Maintain an upright posture and stand back up

Notes and tips:

Aside from working your quads and glutes, dumbbell squats may also provide a good isometric workout for your forearms and upper back, like the farmer's carry.

Dumbbell Sumo Squat

Difficulty: 2

Target muscle:
Quads, Adductors

Secondary muscle(s):
Glutes, hamstrings, lower back

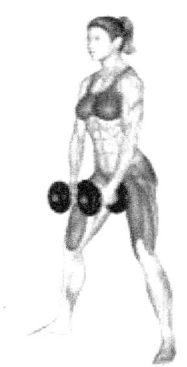 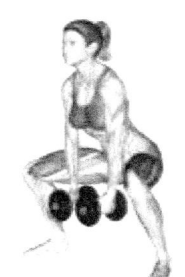

How to:

- Assume a wide stance while holding a pair of dumbbells between your legs. Your feet point outward slightly.

- Tighten your core, inhale, and go down into the squat. Make sure to keep in mind all pointers of a regular body weight squat, which I outlined above

- Maintain an upright posture and stand up into the start position

Notes and tips:

Sumo squats involve the glutes, hamstrings, and adductors to a higher degree than regular squat variations, making them a great hybrid exercise.

For some people, a wider stance feels more comfortable for squatting, so be sure to give this variation a try.

Dumbbell Front Squat

Difficulty: 3

Target muscle:
Quads

Secondary muscle(s):
Abs, glutes, lower back

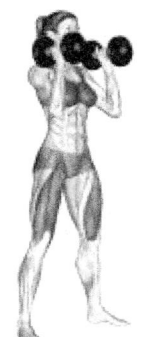
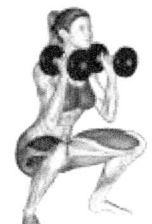

How to:

- Assume a comfortable stance for squatting while holding a pair of dumbbells at shoulder height. You may rest them on your front delts

- Tighten your core, inhale, and go down into the squat. Make sure to keep in mind all pointers of a regular body weight squat from above

- Maintain an upright posture and stand back up into the start position

Notes and tips:

Front squats require more stabilization work from the core and must be performed more upright than a regular squat. Due to the decreased hip involvement, front squats shift the training focus more to the quads and away from the glutes and have your abs work harder than regular squat variations.

However, you may find it more comfortable holding the dumbbells this way instead of at your sides because they can't bump into your legs.

Stair up

Difficulty: 2

Target muscle:
Quads

Secondary muscle(s):
Glutes, lower back

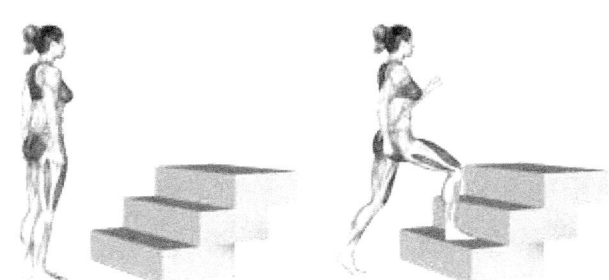

How to:

- Stand in front of a small staircase
- Holding on to the banister, put your right foot on the first step, make sure you have a firm footing, and push yourself up by extending your right knee
- Briefly touch the first step with your left foot
- Bend your right knee slowly and under control until your left foot is firmly planted the floor again
- Complete a set for the right leg, then repeat the exercise for the left

Notes and tips:

As the name suggests, this exercise is highly specific to taking stairs. More advanced individuals may take two steps at a time or hold a dumbbell in their free hand.

Front Foot Elevated Split Squat

Difficulty: 3

Target muscle:
Quads

Secondary muscle(s):
Glutes, lower back

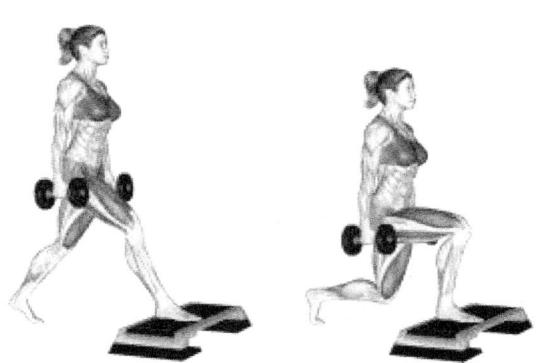

How to:

- Stand in front of a step box or a small staircase and optionally hold a pair of dumbbells
- Put your right foot on the first step and make sure you have a firm footing.
- Keeping an upright torso and a braced core, bend your right leg until your left knee barely touches the floor.
- Reverse the motion and push yourself back up to the start position
- Complete a set for the right leg, then repeat the exercise for the left

Notes and tips:

Taking the next step, if you will, this exercise is a harder variation of the above step ups.

For maximum safety, I would suggest using just one dumbbell and holding on to the banister with your free hand.

Assisted Bulgarian Split Squat

Difficulty: 3

Target muscle:
Quads

Secondary muscle(s):
Glutes, lower back

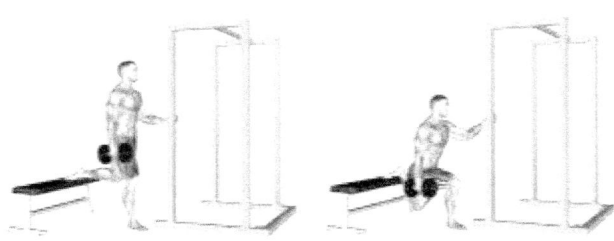

How to:

- Put a chair or workout bench behind you and stand about 2-3 feet in front of it
- While holding a dumbbell, place your left foot on the bench with its sole facing up and make sure you have a firm footing with your right foot.
- Hold on to a stable object or support yourself on a wall with your free hand
- Keeping an upright torso and a braced core, bend your right leg until your thigh is parallel to the floor
- Reverse the motion and push yourself back up into the start position
- Complete a set for the right leg, then repeat the exercise for the left

Notes and tips:

Since this is a single leg exercise that requires lots of strength and stabilization, it is probably only suitable for seniors who have mastered the above squat variations. You can also use these as a glutes and hamstrings exercise if you step out a little further.

Glutes and Hamstrings

I always group glutes and hamstrings together because most hip extension movements work both of these muscle groups, anyway.

Same as the quads, glutes and hamstrings should rank at the top of most seniors' priority list. They are active when we bend over and pick things up from the floor, play a crucial role in relieving the lower back, and support good posture from below.

How to work the glutes and hamstrings:

- Pushing your hips forward with a straight back, either lying down or while being bent over
- Secondarily, the hamstrings also flex the knee joint

Priority: high

Dumbbell Romanian Deadlift

Difficulty: 2

Target muscle:
Hamstrings

Secondary muscle(s):
Glutes, back, forearms, quads

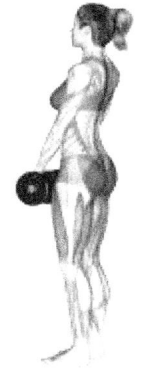
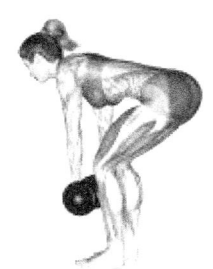

How to:

- Hold a pair of dumbbells in front of your waist and stand about hip-width apart. Your toes may point outward or forward, whichever is more comfortable
- Engage your core and inhale, then slowly bend over from the hips. Push your buttocks back while keeping your chest up to ensure your back stays straight
- As you bend over, keep the dumbbells as close to your body as you can by engaging your lats. You may bend your knees slightly
- Once you feel a good stretch in your hamstrings, reverse the motion to get back into the start position

Notes and tips:

Deadlifts and deadlift variations may seem intimidating at first glance. However, if you do them correctly and perform the movement from the hip instead of the lower back and are careful with your chosen weight, they may yield tons and tons of benefits - chief among them reduced back pain, a strong and stable posterior muscle chain, and lots of carry-over to your everyday life.

Dumbbell Stiff Leg Deadlift

Difficulty: 2

Target muscle:
Hamstrings

Secondary muscle(s):
Glutes, back, forearms

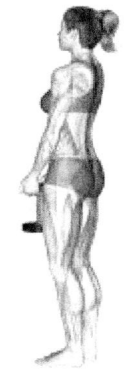
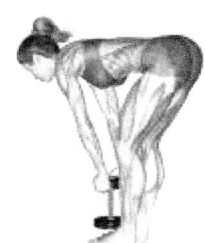

How to:

- Hold a dumbbell in front of your waist and stand about hip-width apart. Your toes may point outwards or forwards, whichever is more comfortable

- Engage your core and inhale, then slowly bend over from the hips. Push your buttocks back while keeping your chest up to ensure your back stays straight

- As you bend over, keep the dumbbells as close to your body as you can by engaging your lats

- Keep your knees as straight as you can

- Once you feel a good stretch in your hamstrings, reverse the motion to get back into the start position

Notes and tips:

These are similar to the Romanian deadlift but since you keep your knees straight, the range of motion is lower.

However, this also means you don't lose tension in the hamstrings, which is good for muscular development. This stretch might also help improve your hamstring flexibility over time and alleviate tightness in that area.

Dumbbell Glute Bridge

Difficulty: 1

Target muscle:
Glutes

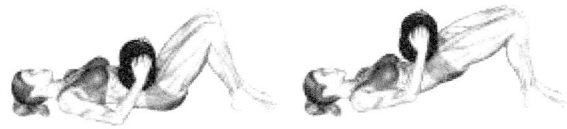

Secondary muscle(s):
Hamstrings

How to:

- Lie down on an exercise mat with bent knees and your feet firmly planted on the floor
- Place a dumbbell onto your abdomen
- Engage your core and inhale, then raise your buttocks off the floor by driving your heels into it.
- In the top position, your thighs and upper body form a straight line
- Hold the tension for a moment, then reverse the motion as you exhale

Notes and tips:

In case lower back issues prevent you from doing any kind of deadlift, glute bridges present an alternative way to strengthen your glutes and hamstrings.

Beginners may want to rest their buttocks on the floor after each repetition or try the exercise with body weight only. If you are more advanced, maintain the tension in your glutes and hamstrings throughout your set. And for the biggest challenge, do the exercise one leg at a time.

Dumbbell Hip Thrust

Difficulty: 2

Target muscle:
Glutes

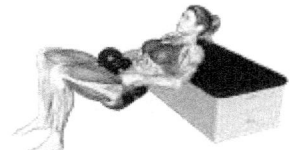 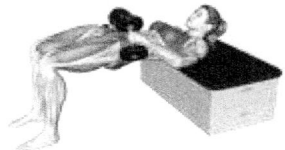

Secondary muscle(s):
Hamstrings

How to:

- Sit down on an exercise mat with your knees bent by 90°. Plant your feet firmly on the floor and rest your upper back against an workout bench or similar elevated surface.

- Make sure this surface is secured against a wall, so it won't move as you perform the exercise

- Hold two dumbbells at your groin, then tighten your core, inhale, and extend your hips. Drive your feet into the floor and your upper back into the bench.

- In the top position, your thighs and upper body should form a straight line

- Hold the tension for a moment, then reverse the motion as you exhale

Notes and tips:

This is an advanced version of our previous exercise and offers more range of motion. Its only drawback is that it requires more effort to set it up.

Dumbbell Lunges

Difficulty: 3

Target muscle:
Glutes

Secondary muscle(s):
Hamstrings, quads

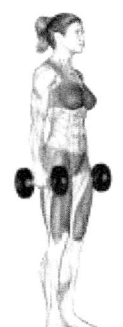 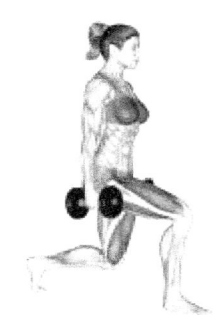

How to:

- While standing, hold a pair of dumbbells at your sides
- Take a wide step forward with your trained leg. This is your start position
- Keeping an upright torso and a braced core, bend your forward leg until your rear knee barely touches the floor.
- Reverse the motion and push yourself back up to the start position
- Complete a set for one leg, then train the other side

Notes and tips:

Like most single leg exercises, lunges might only be suitable for advanced folk. Still, if you have the strength and confidence to do them, I highly recommend you give them a try!

For more stability, you can perform them carrying only one dumbbell and supporting yourself on a wall with your free hand. Just make sure not to lean into it too heavily because this may cause your knee to cave in.

Lying Dumbbell Leg Curl

Difficulty: 2

Target muscle:
Hamstrings

Secondary muscle(s):
--

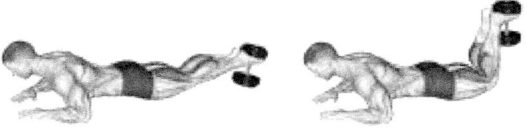

How to:

- Lie prone on an exercise mat
- Grab a dumbbell with your feet (this might require some time to get used to)
- Engage your core and glutes to keep your hips and mid-section stable, then curl the weight up.
- Reverse the motion until you are back in the start position

Notes and tips:

Unless you have access to a gym, it can be tricky to cover knee flexion in your training, the secondary function of your hamstrings.

I admit this exercise might be a bit awkward to do at first, but once you have gotten used to it, it can be a great asset to strengthen your hamstrings.

You may want to be conservative with the dumbbell weight, though. If this exercise is new for you, your hamstrings could easily cramp up when you go too heavy.

Frog Kicks

Difficulty: 2

Target muscle:
Hamstrings

Secondary muscle(s):
--

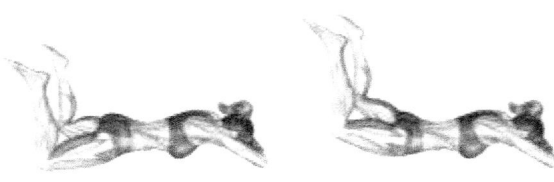

How to:

- Lie prone on an exercise mat with bent knees, so that your soles point to the ceiling. Rest your head on your forearms
- Engage your core and glutes, then push your legs and hips straight up.
- Hold the maximum tension for a moment, then reverse the motion and repeat

Notes and tips:

Frog kicks deliver a great maximum contraction in the glutes. If you have access to an workout bench, consider using it for this exercise to get more range of motion.

Beginners may take a short rest after each repetition, while intermediate and advanced seniors can try to maintain the tension in their glutes and core throughout the set.

Sliding Leg Curl

Difficulty: 3

Target muscle:
Hamstrings

Secondary muscle(s):
Glutes

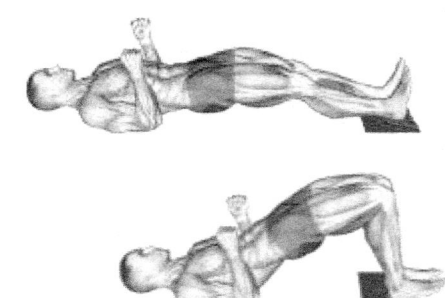

How to:

- Lie stretched out on your back with your feet on a slippery surface, like laminate floor or tile floor.

- Place a towel or cloth between your heels and the floor.

- Create tension in your core and inhale, then drive your heels into the floor so that your buttocks are in the air. Stabilize with your arms

- In the start position, you should rest only on your heels, your arms, and your upper back

- Maintaining tension throughout your body, inhale and then curl your legs towards your buttocks without your hips dropping

- Slowly reverse the motion as you exhale and repeat

Notes and tips:

If you need to make this exercise easier, you can shorten its range of motion. Either start the exercise at its halfway point and curl from there, or curl only halfway up from the bottom.

Calves

The calf muscles, which are called *gastrocnemius* and *soleus*, flex our ankles and are highly active when we walk and run, particularly uphill.

Strong and trained calves don't cramp up as easily, can stabilize the knee from below and are crucial for keeping balance, making it equally crucial to train them properly.

How to work the calves:

- Standing up on your toes

Priority: moderate

Seated Dumbbell Calf Raise

Difficulty: 1

Target muscle:
Calves

Secondary muscle(s):
--

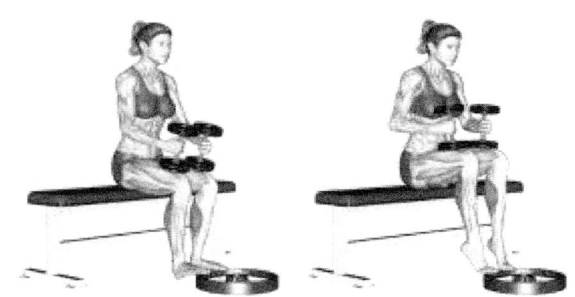

How to:

- Sit down upright on a chair and place a pair of dumbbells onto your thighs
- Place the balls of your feet on an elevated surface
- Toes pointing forwards or slightly outwards, press through the balls of your feet to raise your heels as high as you can
- Hold the tension for a moment in the maximum contracted position, then slowly reverse the motion and repeat

Notes and tips:

It is also okay to do this exercise without placing your feet on an elevated surface, just know that this decreases its effectiveness a bit because you get less range of motion.

You may want to experiment with different toe angles to see which one works best for you, for example: directly to the front, inwards, or outwards.

Standing Calf Raise with Support

Difficulty: 1

Target muscle:
Calves

Secondary muscle(s):
--

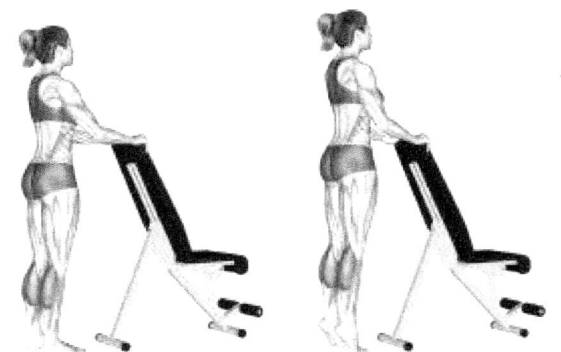

How to:

- Stand hip width apart behind a chair or upright workout bench and hold on to its top
- Toes pointing forwards or slightly outwards, press through the balls of your feet to raise your heels as high as you can
- Hold the tension for a moment in the maximum contracted position, then slowly reverse the motion and repeat

Notes and tips:

With this exercise, the same logic applies as above: to make it more effective, do your calf raises with the balls of your feet on a stable elevated surface to get more range of motion.

If you are up for more of a challenge, consider these variations:

- Standing calf raise without support - do the exercise without holding on to something (optionally even while carrying a pair of dumbbells)
- Single leg calf raise with support - do the exercise one leg at a time

Donkey Calf Raise

Difficulty: 1

Target muscle:
Calves

Secondary muscle(s):
--

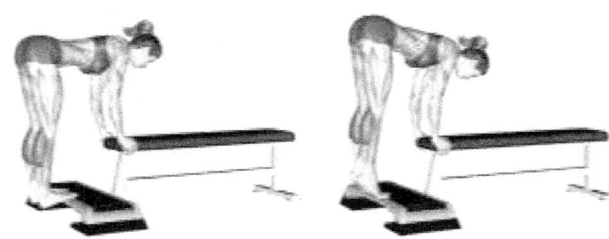

How to:

- Stand hip width apart behind a flat workout bench (or something comparable) on an elevated surface
- Bend forward from the hips and rest your hands on the bench
- Move your feet back to the edge, so that your heels are in the air
- Keeping your knees straight, lower your heels as far as possible until you feel a good stretch
- Press through the balls of your feet to raise your heels as high as you can
- Hold the tension for a moment in the maximum contracted position, then slowly reverse the motion and repeat

Notes and tips:

Donkey calf raises offer a better calf stretch than regular calf raises and eliminate glutes involvement because you don't have to balance yourself.

It is also possible to do these one leg at a time.

Standing Calf Raise on a Staircase

Difficulty: 2

Target muscle:
Calves

Secondary muscle(s):
--

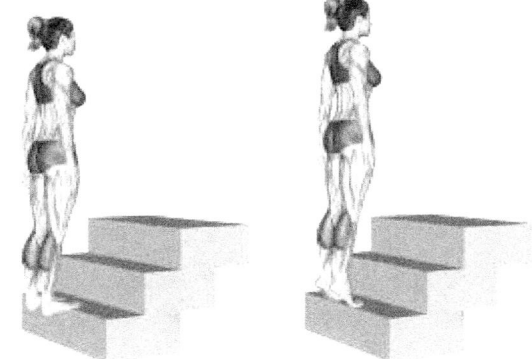

How to:

- Stand hip width apart on the first step of a staircase
- For added safety, hold on to the banister with one hand
- Move your feet back to the edge of the step, so that your heels are in the air
- Keeping your knees straight, lower your heels as far as possible until you feel a good stretch
- Press through the balls of your feet to raise your heels as high as you can
- Hold the tension for a moment in the maximum contracted position, then slowly reverse the motion and repeat

Notes and tips:

As with all standing calf raise variations, consider doing this exercise one leg at a time or while carrying a dumbbell in your free hand.

Example Programs

Let's put our knowledge into practice in some example programs now. I tried to come up with several options, from 2-day-splits to 4-day-splits, so you can find something that fits your schedule and preference. Ideally, you want to spread out your workouts evenly throughout the week to ensure proper recovery. For example, you could train (Mondays + Thursdays), (Tuesdays + Fridays), etc. on a 2-day-split, (Mondays + Wednesdays + Fridays), (Tuesdays + Thursdays + Saturdays), etc. on a 3-day-split and so on.

Just know that although these programs have a general focus (meaning they include all muscle groups), all of them favor legs, hips, back, and shoulders in terms of priority and volume. This simply means that most workouts start with these muscle groups and include more total sets for them than for muscle groups like chest or biceps.

Feel free to pick one of these programs and follow it "as is" or adapt them to your specific needs. In case you go for the latter, know that there aren't any wrong answers, as long as your workout routine is aligned to your goals and abilities, sticks to the programming guidelines of this book, and allows you to be consistent. Don't worry about finding a "perfect" or 100% optimal routine. Go with something that works for you and stick with it.

Templates

To help you find your routine, I first give you my example programs in template form with recommended muscle group orders, set numbers, and repetitions ranges. All you need to do is add exercises from this book to them according to your level of ability.

Repetition ranges

Use the given repetition ranges as guidelines in which you want to get reasonably close to muscle failure. To achieve this, make sure to adapt your dumbbell weights or exercise variations accordingly.

Set numbers

I sometimes give you set ranges in my templates, which are also merely warm recommendations for beginner or intermediate seniors. I would suggest that you start your program with the lower number, wait and see how your body reacts to that workload (i.e. how sore you get), and only add a set here and there in later weeks, in case your workouts get too easy. This should give your body enough time to adapt, without causing too much soreness.

Warmups

Before your working sets, I would suggest having a proper warmup routine in place. If you can spare the time, a few minutes of light cardio (like walking) prior to your workouts helps get the blood flowing into the muscles and mobilize your joints, which is particularly beneficial for leg training. After that, I recommend doing a few test repetitions for each exercise, followed by one or two warmup sets.

For example, let's say you want to do dumbbell rows using 20lbs dumbbells for 10-20 repetitions. A proper warmup could look like this:

- Do 10 rows without weights to loosen your scapulae and shoulders
- Do 8 rows with 10lbs dumbbells (optional)
- Do 5 rows with 20lbs dumbbells
- Do your first working set of 10-20 repetitions.

Rest time between sets

Another common question is how long to rest after a working set. I always go by feel and don't start my next set until I can check four boxes:

- Is my target muscle ready for another set in my repetition range? (For example, the quads for another 10-20 repetitions of squats)
- Are my supporting muscles ready for another set in my repetition range? (For example, the lower back during squats)
- Is my cardiovascular system ready and my breathing normal, so it won't interfere with my set?
- Do I feel psychologically ready for the next set?

Progression

Lastly, I would encourage you to keep a training log to record your workout performances from week to week and occasionally try to beat them by a small margin. Even though progression may not be the main focus in your training, it is still important to slowly but surely get stronger - at least up to a certain point. Of course, rather than "pushing" for progression like someone younger, you may want to let it happen naturally and only do additional reps or add weight without compromising safety. Having a training log may still be helpful in that endeavor because it enables you to keep a long-term overview of your training.

Once you have reached or already are at a strength level you are happy with, you could even shift your focus from progression to mere maintenance. You still keep doing your workouts consistently and train reasonably hard, but instead of going for new records or adding sets, it is also okay for you to maintain your performances and workload over the weeks and months - which also means you maintain your strength.

So, let's examine some programs to see how to get there!

Template 1 - 2-Day-Program

Day 1

Exercise	Sets (Beginners)	Sets (Intermediates)	Repetitions
Quads	2	3-4	10 - 15
Glutes/Hamstrings	2	3-4	8 - 12
Front/Side Delts	2	3-4	10 -15
Back	2	3-4	10 - 20
Chest	1-2	2	12 - 20
Biceps	2	3	12 - 20
Forearms	2	3	12 - 20
Calves	1-2	3	15 - 25
Abs	2	3	10 - 20

Day 2

Exercise	Sets (Beginners)	Sets (Intermediates)	Repetitions
Glutes/Hamstrings	2	3-4	10 - 15
Quads	2	3-4	8 - 12
Back	2	3-4	15 - 20
Front/Side Delts	2	3-4	12 - 20
Chest	1-2	2	10 - 20
Rear Delts	1-2	2	12 - 20
Triceps	1-2	2	15 - 25
Calves	1-2	3	10 - 20
Abs	2	3	10 - 20

Template 2 - 3-Day-Program

Day 1

Exercise	Sets (Beginners)	Sets (Intermediates)	Repetitions
Quads	2	3-4	10 - 20
Glutes/Hamstrings	2	3-4	8 - 12
Front Delts	2	3-4	12 - 20
Chest	1-2	2-3	10 - 20
Side Delts	1-2	2	12 - 20
Calves	1-2	3-4	15 - 25
Abs	1-2	3	10 - 20

Day 2

Exercise	Sets (Beginners)	Sets (Intermediates)	Repetitions
Back	2	3-4	10 -15
Rear Delts	1-2	2-3	10 - 20
Front/Side Delts	2	3-4	10 - 15
Chest	2	3-4	10 - 20
Triceps	1-2	2-3	15 - 25
Biceps	2	3-4	15 - 25

Day 3

Exercise	Sets (Beginners)	Sets (Intermediates)	Repetitions
Glutes/Hamstrings	2	2-3	10 - 15
Quads	2	2-3	8 - 12
Glutes/Hamstrings	1-2	2-3	10 - 20
Quads	1-2	2-3	10 - 20
Calves	1-2	2-3	12 - 20
Back	2	3-4	15 - 20
Forearms	1-2	3	12 - 20
Abs	1-2	3	10 - 20

Template 3 - 4-Day-Program

Day 1

Exercise	Sets (Beg.)	Sets (Int.)	Repetitions
Front Delts	2	3	8 - 12
Side Delts	2	3	10 - 20
Back	2	3-4	10 - 20
Rear Delts	1-2	2-3	12 - 20
Chest	1-2	2-3	10 - 20
Forearms	1-2	2-3	15 - 25
Biceps	1-2	3	10 - 20

Day 2

Exercise	Sets (Beg.)	Sets (Int.)	Repetitions
Quads	2	3-4	8 - 12
Glutes/Hamstrings	2	3-4	10 - 20
Calves	2	3-4	10 - 15
Abs	2	3-4	10 - 20

Day 3

Exercise	Sets (Beg.)	Sets (Int.)	Repetitions
Back	2	3-4	8 - 12
Rear Delts	2	2-3	10 - 20
Front Delts	1-2	3-4	10 - 20
Side Delts	1-2	3-4	10 - 20
Chest	1-2	2-3	12 - 20
Forearms	2	2-3	10 - 15
Triceps	1-2	2-3	12 - 20

Day 4

Exercise	Sets (Beg.)	Sets (Int.)	Repetitions
Glutes/Hamstrings	2	3-4	8 - 12
Quads	2	3-4	10 - 20
Calves	2	3-4	12 - 20
Abs	2	3-4	10 - 15

2-Day Beginner Program (without bench)

Day 1

Exercise	Page	Sets	Repetitions
Dumbbell Bench Squat	92	2	10 - 15
Dumbbell Glute Bridge	104	2	8 - 12
Seated Dumbbell Shoulder Press	28	2	12 - 20
Bent Over Dumbbell Row	44	2	10 -15
Kneeling Push-ups	58	1	10 - 20
Seated Biceps Curls	63	2	12 - 20
Farmer's Carry	78	2	20-40 seconds
Seated Calf Raises	111	2	15 - 25
Quarter Sit-ups	82	2	10 - 20

Day 2

Exercise	Page	Sets	Repetitions
Dumbbell Romanian Deadlift	102	2	10 - 15
Stair up	98	2 per leg	8 - 12
One-Arm Dumbbell Row	46	2 per arm	15 - 20
Dumbbell Side Lateral Raises	33	2	12 - 20
Incline Push-ups	59	1	10 - 20
Bent Over Face Pull	38	2	12 - 20
Dumbbell Triceps Extension	68	1	15 - 25
Standing Calf Raise with Support	112	2	10 - 20
Bottoms up	85	2	10 - 20

2-Day Beginner Program (with bench)

Day 1

Exercise	Page	Sets	Repetitions
Dumbbell Bench Squat	92	2	10 - 15
Dumbbell Glute Bridge	104	2	8 - 12
Incline Dumbbell Shoulder Press	30	2	12 - 20
Incline Dumbbell Row	47	2	10 - 15
Dumbbell Bench Press	51	1	10 - 20
Seated Biceps Curls	63	2	12 - 20
Farmer's Carry	78	2	20-40 seconds
Seated Calf Raises	111	2	15 - 25
Quarter Sit-ups	82	2	10 - 20

Day 2

Exercise	Page	Sets	Repetitions
Dumbbell Romanian Deadlift	102	2	10 - 15
Stair up	98	2 per leg	8 - 12
One-Arm Dumbbell Row	46	2 per arm	15 - 20
Dumbbell Side Lateral Raises	33	2	12 - 20
Incline Dumbbell Bench Press	52	1	10 - 20
Incline Rear Delt Fly	40	2	12 - 20
Incline Triceps Extension	69	1	15 - 25
Standing Calf Raise with Support	112	2	10 - 20
Bottoms up	85	2	10 - 20

3-Day Beginner Program (without bench)

Day 1

Exercise	Page	Sets	Repetitions
Dumbbell Bench Squat	92	2	10 - 20
Dumbbell Glute Bridge	104	2	8 - 12
Seated Dumbbell Shoulder Press	28	2	12 - 20
Kneeling Push-ups	58	1	10 - 20
Dumbbell Side Lateral Raises	33	1	12 - 20
Seated Calf Raises	111	2	15 - 25
Quarter Sit-ups	82	2	10 - 20

Day 2

Exercise	Page	Sets	Repetitions
Bent Over Dumbbell Row	44	2	10 - 15
Seated Rear Delt Fly	39	1	10 - 20
Seated Front Raise	31	2	10 - 15
Dumbbell Side Lateral Raise	33	2	10 - 20
Wall Push-ups	60	2	15 - 25
Dumbbell Triceps Extension	68	1	15 - 25
Seated Biceps Curls	63	2	10 - 15

Day 3

Exercise	Page	Sets	Repetitions
Dumbbell Romanian Deadlift	102	2	10 - 15
Dumbbell Wall Squat	94	2	8 - 12
Standing Calf Raise with Support	112	2	12 - 20
One-Arm Dumbbell Row	46	2 per arm	15 - 20
Farmer's Carry	78	2	20 - 40 seconds
Bottoms up	85	2	10 - 20

3-Day Beginner Program (with bench)

Day 1

Exercise	Page	Sets	Repetitions
Dumbbell Bench Squat	93	2	10 - 20
Dumbbell Glute Bridge	104	2	8 - 12
Seated Dumbbell Shoulder Press	28	2	12 - 20
Dumbbell Bench Press	51	1	10 - 20
Dumbbell Side Lateral Raises	33	1	12 - 20
Seated Calf Raises	111	2	15 - 25
Quarter Sit-ups	82	2	10 - 20

Day 2

Exercise	Page	Sets	Repetitions
Bent Over Dumbbell Row	44	2	10 -15
Incline Rear Delt Fly	40	1	10 - 20
Arnold Press	29	2	10 - 15
Incline Dumbbell Bench Press	52	2	10 - 20
Incline Triceps Extension	69	1	15 - 25
Prone Incline Curls	65	2	15 - 25

Day 3

Exercise	Page	Sets	Repetitions
Dumbbell Romanian Deadlift	102	2	10 - 15
Dumbbell Wall Squat	94	2	8 - 12
Standing Calf Raise with Support	112	2	12 - 20
Incline Dumbbell Row	47	2	15 - 20
Farmer's Carry	78	2	20 - 40 seconds
Bottoms up	85	2	10 - 20

3-Day Intermediate Program (without bench)

Day 1

Exercise	Page	Sets	Repetitions
Dumbbell Squat	95	3	10 - 20
Dumbbell Glute Bridge	104	3	8 - 12
Arnold Press	29	3	12 - 20
Incline Push-ups	59	2	10 - 20
Dumbbell Side Lateral Raises	33	2	12 - 20
Seated Calf Raises	111	3	15 - 25
Quarter Sit-ups	82	3	10 - 20

Day 2

Exercise	Page	Sets	Repetitions
Bent Over Dumbbell Row	44	3	10 -15
Seated Rear Delt Fly	39	2	10 - 20
Seated Dumbbell Shoulder Press	28	3	10 - 15
Dumbbell Floor Press	56	2	10 - 20
Floor Flys	55	2	15 - 25
Dumbbell Triceps Extension	68	2	15 - 25
Seated Biceps Curls	63	3	10 - 15

Day 3

Exercise	Page	Sets	Repetitions
Dumbbell Romanian Deadlift	102	3	10 - 15
Dumbbell Front Squat	97	3	8 - 12
Frog Kicks	108	2	10 - 20
Body Weight Squat	90	2	10 - 20
Donkey Calf Raise	113	3	12 - 20
One-Arm Dumbbell Row	46	3 per arm	15 - 20
Suitcase Carry	79	2 per arm	30 - 60 seconds
Bottoms up	85	2	10 - 20

3-Day Intermediate Program (with bench)

Day 1

Exercise	Page	Sets	Repetitions
Dumbbell Squat	95	3	10 - 20
Dumbbell Hip Thrust	105	3	8 - 12
Arnold Press	29	3	12 - 20
Dumbbell Bench Press	51	2	10 - 20
Dumbbell Side Lateral Raises	33	2	12 - 20
Seated Calf Raises	111	3	15 - 25
Quarter Sit-ups	82	3	10 - 20

Day 2

Exercise	Page	Sets	Repetitions
Bent Over Dumbbell Row	44	3	10 -15
Incline Rear Delt Fly	40	2	10 - 20
Seated Dumbbell Shoulder Press	28	3	10 - 15
Incline Dumbbell Bench Press	52	2	10 - 20
Hyght Dumbbell Flys	54	2	15 - 25
Incline Triceps Extension	69	2	15 - 25
Prone Incline Curls	65	3	10 - 15

Day 3

Exercise	Page	Sets	Repetitions
Dumbbell Romanian Deadlift	102	3	10 - 15
Dumbbell Front Squat	97	3	8 - 12
Frog Kicks	108	2	10 - 20
Dumbbell Bench Squat	93	2	10 - 20
Donkey Calf Raise	113	3	12 - 20
One-Arm Dumbbell Row	46	3 per arm	15 - 20
Suitcase Carry	79	2 per arm	30 - 60 seconds
Bottoms up	85	2	10 - 20

4-Day Intermediate Program (without bench)

Day 1

Exercise	Page	Sets	Repetitions
Seated Dumbbell Shoulder Press	28	3	8 - 12
Dumbbell Side Lateral Raise	33	3	10 - 20
One-Arm Dumbbell Row	46	3	10 - 20
Lying Prone Ws	48	2	12 - 20
Floor Press	56	3	10 - 20
Reverse Curls	75	2	15 - 25
Cross-Body Hammer Curls	77	3	10 - 20

Day 2

Exercise	Page	Sets	Repetitions
Dumbbell Squat	95	4	8 - 12
Dumbbell Stiff Leg Deadlift	103	4	10 - 20
Donkey Calf Raise	113	4	10 - 15
Twisting Crunch	84	4	10 - 20

Day 3

Exercise	Page	Sets	Repetitions
Bent Over Dumbbell Rows	44	3	8 - 12
Bent Over Face Pull	38	2	10 - 20
Seated Front Raise	31	3	10 - 20
W-Press	36	3	10 - 20
Push-ups	57	3	10 - 20
Behind the Back Finger Curls	76	3	10 - 15
Dumbbell Triceps Extensions	68	3	15 - 25

Day 4

Exercise	Page	Sets	Repetitions
Dumbbell Glute Bridge	104	4	8 - 12
Dumbbell Front Squat	97	4	10 - 20
Seated Calf Raises	111	4	12 - 20
Hip Lift	86	4	10 - 20

4-Day Intermediate Program (with bench)

Day 1

Exercise	Page	Sets	Repetitions
Seated Dumbbell Shoulder Press	28	3	8 - 12
Dumbbell Side Lateral Raise	33	3	10 - 20
One-Arm Dumbbell Row	46	3	10 - 20
Incline Y-Raise	41	2	12 - 20
Dumbbell Bench Press	51	3	10 - 20
Reverse Curls	75	2	15 - 25
Prone Incline Curls	65	3	10 - 20

Day 2

Exercise	Page	Sets	Repetitions
Dumbbell Squat	95	4	8 - 12
Dumbbell Stiff Leg Deadlift	103	4	10 - 20
Donkey Calf Raise	113	4	10 - 15
Twisting Crunch	84	4	10 - 20

Day 3

Exercise	Page	Sets	Repetitions
Incline Dumbbell Row	47	3	8 - 12
Incline Rear Delt Fly	40	2	10 - 20
Incline Front Raise	32	3	10 - 20
W-Press	36	3	10 - 20
Incline Dumbbell Bench Press	52	3	10 - 20
Behind the Back Finger Curls	76	3	10 - 15
Dumbbell Incline French Press	70	3	15 - 25

Day 4

Exercise	Page	Sets	Repetitions
Dumbbell Hip Thrust	105	4	8 - 12
Dumbbell Front Squat	97	4	10 - 20
Seated Calf Raises	111	4	12 - 20
Forward Step Front Plank	88	4	10 - 20

Adapting and Developing a Program

Again, the above are merely examples of what a decent program may look like. Feel free to mix-and-match and adapt these in any way you see fit. For example, you may pick other exercises for the same muscle groups, use slightly different set numbers, change the exercise order according to your training goals, or do two exercises instead of just one for a muscle group (i.e. instead of four sets of dumbbell squats for your quads, you do just two sets of dumbbell squats followed by two sets of front squats).

The important thing is that you feel like there is something "going on" in your muscles after your workouts, like moderate wonkiness and soreness. However, make sure it doesn't get too extreme or painful and avoid doing "too much" right from the start. This is also the main reason why I advise you to begin your program with conservative set numbers and take it from there. Once you get the feeling that your workload for a specific muscle is too small, despite training reasonably hard, consider adding a set here and there or switch to a more challenging exercise variation. Take your soreness and exhaustion as gauges and base your decisions to "do more work" on them. For complete beginners, this could eventually mean switching from a 2-day plan to a 3-day plan to keep their workout length reasonable. That said, at the end of the day, strength training is all about personal preference. As long as your volume needs are covered, you exert reasonable effort, and gradually get stronger (or at least maintain your strength), it won't matter whether you do shorter, more frequent workouts or longer, less frequent workouts.

What matters is that you keep training consistently to stay strong, healthy, and independent until your last day on this earth - which, hopefully, will still be a long time coming.

Conclusion

All right, I think it is time to wrap up this book, so you can finally get started!

From the bottom of my heart, I hope that these training tips, programs, and exercises will help you improve your quality of life. Remember, not everyone has the courage or the will to change their situation for the better or to take measures early on to prevent issues that are tied to old age. Let me once again thank you for buying this book and rest assured that I wish you nothing but the best for your health and your future.

If you found the contents of this book useful, would you mind my asking you again to leave a short review? This way you could tell other people your age about your experiences and help them with their purchase decision.

Take care!

Yours truly,

Andy

References

1. Effects of resistance training on older adults
https://pubmed.ncbi.nlm.nih.gov/15107011/

2. The effect of resistance training on cognitive function in the older adults: a systematic review of randomized clinical trials
https://pubmed.ncbi.nlm.nih.gov/30006762/

3. Effects of resistance training on functional ability in elderly individuals
https://pubmed.ncbi.nlm.nih.gov/21361808/

4. The effects of resistance training on well-being and memory in elderly volunteers
https://pubmed.ncbi.nlm.nih.gov/9884004/

5. Effect of resistance training set volume on upper body muscle hypertrophy: are more sets really better than less?
https://pubmed.ncbi.nlm.nih.gov/29024332/

6. Training volume landmarks for muscle growth
https://rpstrength.com/training-volume-landmarks-muscle-growth/

7. Training Frequency For Muscle Growth: What The Data Say
https://www.strongerbyscience.com/frequency-muscle/

8. Influence of Resistance Training Proximity-to-Failure on Skeletal Muscle Hypertrophy: A Systematic Review with Meta-analysis
https://pubmed.ncbi.nlm.nih.gov/36334240/

9. Effects of Low- vs. High-Load Resistance Training on Muscle Strength and Hypertrophy in Well-Trained Men
https://pubmed.ncbi.nlm.nih.gov/25853914/

10. Progressing for Hypertrophy
https://rpstrength.com/expert-advice/progressing-for-hypertrophy

11. Exercise training guidelines for the elderly
https://pubmed.ncbi.nlm.nih.gov/9927004/

12. Size, Strength, and Ageing
https://www.youtube.com/watch?v=r8zcF6Ut7lo

All illustrations used in this book were downloaded from gymvisual.com and are licensed under account andreas.taumann@web.de

Printed in Dunstable, United Kingdom